CANADIAN MEDICAL LIVES NO. 17

R.G. FERGUSON

Crusader Against Tuberculosis

To L. Randy Brown
with warm personal
regards

C. Stuart Houston

C. STUART HOUSTON

Series Editor: T.P. Morley

Hannah Institute
&
Dundurn Press
Toronto and Oxford
1991

Editing: Leslie Derbecker
Cover Design: JAQ
Page Design and Production: Karen Dahlstrom
Printing and Binding: Gagné Printing Ltd., Louiseville, Quebec, Canada

The writing of this manuscript and the publication of this book were made possible by support from several sources. The publisher wishes to acknowledge the generous assistance and ongoing support of **The Canada Council, The Book Publishing Industry Development Programme of the Department of Communications** and **The Ontario Arts Council.**

J. Kirk Howard, Publisher

Canadian Cataloguing in Publication Data

Houston, C. Stuart (Clarence Stuart), 1927-
R.G. Ferguson: crusader against tuberculosis

(Canadian medical lives ; no. 17)
Co-published by the Hannah Institute for the History of Medicine.
Includes bibliographical references and index.
ISBN 1-55002-143-5

1. Ferguson, R.G. (Robert George), 1883-1964.
2. Tuberculosis – Saskatchewan. 3. Saskatchewan Anti-Tuberculosis League – Biography. 4. Physicians – Canada – Biography. I. Hannah Institute for the History of Medicine. II. Title. III. Series.

RA644.T7H6 1991 616.9'95'0092 C91-095291-4

Dundurn Press Limited
2181 Queen Street East
Suite 301
Toronto, Canada
M4E 1E5

Dundurn Distribution Limited
73 Lime Walk
Headington
Oxford, England
OX3 7AD

CANADIAN MEDICAL LIVES SERIES

The story of the Hannah Institute for the History of Medicine has been told by John B. Neilson and G.R. Paterson in *Associated Medical Services, Incorporated: A History* (1987). With the creation of the Institute the AMS endowed it with funds, capability and responsibility to develop and disseminate a body of medical history hitherto hidden in the country's memory.

A grants and personnel support program enables the Institute through medical, social and political historians to become a powerful influence in the rapidly expanding interest accorded to medical history. A chair in the history of medicine is supported at each of the five Ontario medical schools. Originally the Institute's support was limited to Ontario, but it has now been extended to medical historical work in any part of Canada.

Dr. Donald R. Wilson, President of Associated Medical Services, persuaded the Board that the Hannah Institute should launch a series of biographies of those who, as yet unsung, had made major contributions in the broad field of Canadian medicine during their lifetime. The Institute also had in mind for the series members of the nursing profession, particularly those who had pioneered public health services, as well as workers in related fields.

Stuart Houston lives in Ferguson's Saskatchewan and knows many of his family and contemporaries, but his admiration for Ferguson does not stand in the way of objectivity. He writes of one man's triumph in mobilizing a province against the scourge of tuberculosis. As a public health venture it was a success, not diminished by the arrival of chemotherapy which rendered the program obsolete. Ferguson's scientific and epidemiological planning is part history, but the example of his tenacity endures.

The next volumes in the Canadian Medical Lives Series include Maude Abbot (Douglas Waugh), Earle Scarlett (F.W. Musselwhite), J.C.B. Grant (C.L.N. Robinson), Harold Griffith (Richard Bodman and Deirdre Gillies), Mahlon W. Locke (Robert Jackson) and William Boyd (Ian Carr).

There is no shortage of meritorious subjects. Willing and capable authors are difficult to acquire. The Institute is therefore deeply grateful to the early authors who have already committed their time and skill to the series.

T.P. Morley
Series Editor
1991

CANADIAN MEDICAL LIVES SERIES

1. *Duncan Graham* by Robert B. Kerr and Douglas Waugh*
2. *Bill Mustard* by Marilyn Dunlop*
3. *Joe Doupe* by Terence Moore*
4. *Clarence Hincks* by Charles G. Roland*
5. *Francis A.C. Scrimger, V.C.,* by Suzanne Kingsmill*
6. *Emily Stowe* by Mary Beacock Fryer*
7. *William Canniff* by Heather MacDougall
8. *Harold Griffith* by Richard Bodman and Deirdre Gillies
9. *Earle P. Scarlett* by F.W. Musselwhite*
10. *Marguerite Carr-Harris, RN,* by Meryn Stuart
11. *Mahlon W. Locke* by Robert Jackson
12. *Wallace Graham* by Joan Hollobon
13. *Maude Abbott* by Douglas Waugh
14. *J.C.B. Grant* by C.L.N. Robinson
15. *William Boyd* by Ian Carr
16. *William Carson* by H.H. Nixon
17. *R.G. Ferguson* by C. Stuart Houston*
18. *William T. Aikins* by Charles M. Godfrey
19. *Brock Chisholm* by Allan Irving

* published

CANADIAN MEDICAL LIVES NO. 17

R.G. FERGUSON

Crusader Against Tuberculosis

C. STUART HOUSTON

Series Editor: T.P. Morley

TABLE OF CONTENTS

ACKNOWLEDGEMENTS

I AM INDEBTED to the Ferguson clan for allowing my wife Mary and me, the only outsiders, to attend their weekend reunion at Kindersley, Saskatchewan, at the end of July 1988. I interviewed many members of the extended family and was able to ascertain the location and extent of the manuscripts and memorabilia so freely shared in the year that followed.

I am grateful to Dr. Robert Ferguson and his wife Norma for their hospitality at Fort Qu'Appelle, and permission to copy his father's student account books and boyhood reminiscences; to Patricia (Ferguson) Motherwell-Dyck for many helpful and detailed letters; to Sheelagh (Ferguson) Barrable for poems, reminiscences, a copy of her father's diary of his canoe trip to La Loche, and details on the Mickle Fellowship; to Margaret (Ferguson) Fallis for her hospitality in Victoria, British Columbia; to Dr. David B. Stewart and his wife Ruth for their hospitality at Killarney, for access to the bound volumes of his father's writings, and for a guided tour of the buildings remaining at Ninette Sanatorium; to Mrs. Nancy Smith for the Ferguson genealogy; to Helen Williams for the Margaret Jane Ferguson obituary; and to Maxine and Marvin Wilson of Joliette, North Dakota, who provided homestead maps and depositions and a historical booklet of the Joliette United Methodist Church, and who gave us a guided tour of the Ferguson homestead.

Dr. Brian Graham, executive director of the Saskatchewan Lung Association, provided free access to the original minutes of the Saskatchewan Anti-tuberculosis League and to a complete set of bound volumes of the *Valley Echo*; Darcy Hande, Saskatchewan Archives, allowed perusal of a microfilm copy of the minutes of the Saskatchewan Association of Rural Municipalities, a nearly complete version of which was consulted further in *Western Municipal News* in Special Collections, University of Saskatchewan Library, accessed with the aid of Shirley Martin; Mrs. Ann Bilodeau and Dr. D.C. Mortimer placed much archival material at my disposal in the National Research Council Archives, Ottawa; Dr. Jack D. Key made many early books and journals available in the Mayo Clinic Library, Rochester, Minnesota; Audrey Kerr made available the David A. Stewart papers and bibliography in the University of Manitoba Medical Library; Dr. Wilma Sweaney and her staff provided access to the D.M. Baltzan and Brodie collections of medical history in the Health Sciences Library, University of Saskatchewan; Darlene E. Hamilton at the Seattle Public Library provided a biographical sketch of David Ferguson and transcriptions from Polk's city directories for Bellingham and Seattle, Washington; and G.W. Jensen, Yorkton city clerk, provided details concerning the burial plot of Margaret Jane Ferguson.

Two drafts of this book were read and criticized by Mary I. Houston and Margaret Belcher. The initial draft was also read and criticized by J. Frank Roy; Dr. Stanley C. Houston; Dr. David B. Stewart; Dr. Vern Hoeppner; Dr. G.D. Barnett, former medical superintendent of the Saskatchewan Anti-tuberculosis League; Dr. Brian Graham and Ken More of the Saskatchewan Lung Association; Dr. James A. Dosman; Dr. Anne Fanning; Dr. Robert Ferguson; Sheelagh (Ferguson) Barrable and her son, Bill Barrable; Patricia (Ferguson) Motherwell-Dyck; Margaret (Ferguson) Fallis; and David Ferguson. Mrs. Joan Matlock helped me enter revisions into the word processor. I am grateful for many helpful comments, but if any errors persist, they are my responsibility alone.

CSH
Saskatoon, Saskatchewan
1991

FOREWORD

THE LATE DR. Geoffrey Bilson observed that medical history has usually been written by medical doctors: "This has resulted in an emphasis on biography and a tendency to see the history of medicine as a history of progress brought about by individuals." I see myself as a biographer of this persuasion rather than as a social historian who "tends to put less emphasis on individual achievements and more emphasis on broader social developments," making "medical history less self-congratulatory."

This book tells the story of a medical doctor, George Ferguson, who made things happen, who mobilized and taught and inspired an entire province. It is also the story of tuberculosis in Saskatchewan.

My mother, Sigga Christianson, a final-year medical student at the University of Manitoba, worked at the Fort Qu'Appelle Sanatorium the summer before she graduated. Ferguson had made a profound impression on her and, even now, in her ninety-eighth year, her countenance brightens up whenever I mention Dr. Ferguson. Mother was one of the "doctors" involved in the tuberculosis survey of Weyburn school children in 1924, which at the time was considered an important "first." Instead of the usual compulsory two weeks of tuberculosis training, Mother was at the San from the first of May until the end of September in 1924, and her official transcript shows that, in return for her extra time at the San, she received full credit for four months of internal medicine. Many times she has said she worshipped the ground that Ferguson walked on.

As a young and impressionable lad I knew Dr. Ferguson well. He came to luncheon at our home each time he took the monthly tuberculosis clinic at the Yorkton hospital. My father, the late Dr. Clarence J. Houston of Yorkton, enjoyed Ferguson's company immensely and saw him often. My father's sister, Mary Houston, was a registered nurse who worked several stints at the San, both before and after she returned to the family farm near Tyvan, Saskatchewan, to look after her ageing mother. In later years she was matron in charge of one of the pavilions and, each May twenty-fourth, was the first at the San to take a "dip" in the lake.

There were other connections. The Ferguson farm was just south of Yorkton and Ferguson's mother and his sister, Mrs. Mel Ruttle, who lived ten miles west of Yorkton, were patients of my parents. I read the jokes in the monthly *Valley Echo*, the sanatorium newsmagazine, and I often listened to the weekly amateur hour on CJGX radio, which raised extra funds for the Anti-tuberculosis League. I went to Boy Scout summer camp between Lebret and Fort Qu'Appelle, on the former property of Dr. Seymour, the man instrumental in starting the Anti-tuberculosis League and in choosing the site of the sanatorium. My classmate John More and I chose Fort Qu'Appelle for our two weeks of compulsory tuberculosis training at the end of our fourth year in 1950. My father was an honorary pallbearer at Ferguson's funeral. More recently, I placed aluminum leg bands on two nestling bald eagles on the island named for Dr. Ferguson, the largest island in Montreal Lake.

In 1986, three chance events ordained that I should write this book. Dr. Ian Carr, editor of *Manitoba Medicine*, asked me to write a "reminiscence" of my student days. What would I write about? What had changed most? Tuberculosis teaching. I wrote "Reminiscences: compulsory tuberculosis training for Manitoba medical students." Two generations of students, including both my parents and myself, in the Manitoba classes of 1925, 1926 and 1951, had been required to obtain two weeks of practical experience at a tuberculosis sanatorium. Next I went to the annual meeting of the Royal College of Physicians and Surgeons in Toronto. My son, Dr. Stanley C. Houston, a Fellow in infectious diseases at the University of Alberta, gave a paper on the use of BCG in the prevention of tuberculosis. To my astonishment he told the medical audience that Ferguson's original studies of BCG among Indians and student nurses were the best constructed of many such studies ever done. The third event was a call from the dean of medicine, Dr. Ian McDonald. The Hannah Foundation for the History of Medicine had asked whether any Saskatchewan doctor merited inclusion in a new series of Canadian medical biographies. Did I know of such a doctor, and if so, who could write his biography? As a final coincidence, I was due for a year's sabbatical leave. I capitulated and volunteered.

MY FATHER

Discerning thinker,
Accurately concise,
Seeking truth,
Displaying courage,
Inspiring others.

Wise administrator,
Patient diplomat,
Intensely dedicated,
Endearingly modest,
Quietly conspicuous.

Perceptive physician,
Tireless researcher,
Prolonging life,
Alleviating pain,
Renewing hope.

Loving father,
Understanding frailties,
Encouraging initiative,
Stimulating faith,
Teaching humility,
My Father.

Sheelagh (Ferguson) Barrable,
on Father's Day, June 1959

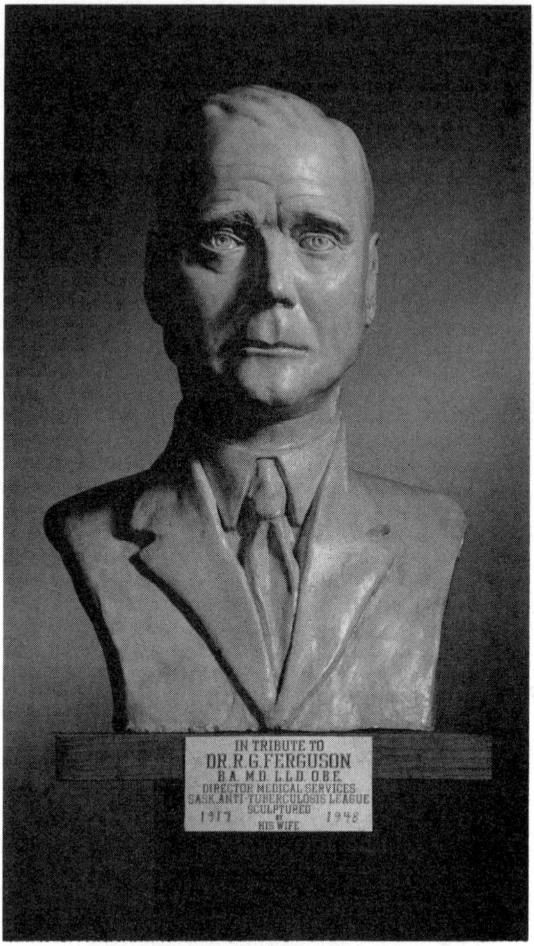
IN TRIBUTE TO
DR. R. G. FERGUSON
B.A. M.D. L.L.D. O.B.E.
DIRECTOR MEDICAL SERVICES
SASK. ANTI-TUBERCULOSIS LEAGUE
SCULPTURED
BY
HIS WIFE
1917
1948

Bust of Dr. R. G. Ferguson, sculpted by his wife.

— Chapter One —

Education

Boyhood, 1883 –1901

ROBERT GEORGE FERGUSON was born on 12 September 1883 on the family farm at South Joliette, North Dakota, only seventeen miles south of the Canadian boundary, about sixty miles north of Grand Forks. To avoid confusion with his father, Robert Ferguson, the family used the lad's second name, George.

George's grandfather, James Ferguson, had been born in Ireland in 1814 near Moy, County Tyrone, on the west bank of the Blackwater River, south of Lough Neagh. James had emigrated to Ontario in 1839, but the first of his three wives, Frances Ellis, and three daughters had died on the ocean crossing during an epidemic, probably from cholera. James remarried, this time to Frances Hunt. When she died, Ferguson, at sixty-four, married his seventeen-year-old hired girl, Frances Jordan, and had another seven children. James Ferguson died in 1902 at Glen Huron, Ontario.

Robert Ferguson, George's father, was the oldest of the eight children of James Ferguson's second marriage. Robert was born on a farm in Carleton County southwest of Ottawa, Ontario, on 16 August 1850. When he was six his parents moved to Kincardine township, Bruce County, near the banks of Lake Huron.

George's mother, Margaret Jane Fisher, was born on 7 June 1855 between Bervie and Ripley in Kincardine Township. Her parents had died of tuberculosis before she was seven years of age, and she was raised by her older sister. James Ferguson, fearing the history of tuberculosis in the Fisher family, opposed Robert's marriage to Margaret Jane, so the young couple eloped on 15 July 1874. After six years of marriage and three children, Margaret Jane's health began to fail. Knowledge of the family history of tuberculosis may have played a part in the local doctor's advice to the young couple to move west. The prospects appeared better for Robert as well, for their Ontario farm was heavily wooded and clearing was slow. In 1881 they moved to North Dakota.

George was the sixth in a family of sixteen (one a stillborn twin) born to Robert and Margaret Jane Ferguson. The births of the fourth to eighth Ferguson children in their North Dakota farm home were not registered in the state capital at Bismarck. Years later, this omission caused George Ferguson endless trouble as a Canadian citizen born in the United States, unable to prove when or where he had been born. Matters were finally settled by obtaining an affidavit from his mother, together with a copy of the entries of all the children's births in the family bible.

Robert Ferguson farmed 480 acres in Township 161 north, Range 51 west of the Fifth Principal Meridian, located just over a mile west of the Red River, and three miles south and one mile east of the village of Joliette.[1]

Joliette was named for a community of the same name in the province of Quebec, from which some of the early settlers had come. Contrary to Ferguson family legend, it was not named for Father Louis Joliet, the famous explorer who, with Father Jacques Marquette and five companions, discovered that the Mississippi River flowed into the Gulf of Mexico and not into the Pacific Ocean.

Although his Orangeman father bore scars on his back resulting from a Catholic ambush before he left Ireland, Robert was on the best of terms with his Catholic neighbours, among them Ernest Pariseau, a friend with whom he shared mutual understanding and trust. The Roman Catholic and Methodist churches in Joliette were side by side and the congregations attended each other's social functions. Nevertheless, each maintained its own customs, such as shivarees and wakes, and the Orangemen held a Protestant parade every 12 July.

Robert Ferguson's closest friend was James McCauley, a big, good-hearted Irishman. For fifteen years the Ferguson and McCauley families went back and forth to celebrate Christmas and New Year's together – and backed each other's notes at the bank.

George fortunately left written reminiscences of his early days on the farm. He described his mother as a tall, beautiful, striking woman with black hair, blue eyes and milk-white skin. A good conversationalist, she spoke softly and deliberately. She carried herself with poise and dignity. A voracious reader, religious, even-tempered and hospitable, she was able to make anyone feel at ease. Although somewhat delicate, she worked hard and rarely hired any help in raising her fifteen children.

Mrs. Ferguson was a postmistress for four or five years. The stage coach from Pembina to Grand Forks stopped to drop mail at the rural post office, named South Joliette, on the Ferguson farm. Often meals were served to stagecoach passengers.

Robert was a witty, kindly, generous man with a very quick temper. A singer and a talented conversationalist, he enjoyed a battle of wits. He was a teetotaller and non-smoker. Scrupulously honest, his word was as good as his bond. He took out American citizenship papers and voted Democrat. Though poor, Robert Ferguson supported the church and looked after the needy.

There were good times and bad times. George wrote later of the "barn-raising bee" on their farm. One summer a cyclone struck their granary and destroyed their fanning mill. The same year there was a raffle, with a fanning mill as the prize. His mother, quite against her principles, bought a raffle ticket and was the lucky winner.

When George was four, his eleven-year-old brother Thomas, the eldest and the family favourite, was killed. Three different versions of the event have been passed down through the family. One that he fell off a wagon and the wheel ran over his head; the second, that he fell from a stoneboat when the horses bolted; the third had Thomas helping the hired man shovel frozen manure from the barn on to a sleigh, when a large frozen lump fell from the top of the pile and struck his head. When a new baby brother arrived the next month, on 2 May 1887, he was also christened Thomas, because the dead boy had been so endearing, helpful and thoughtful. Earlier in that pregnancy the older Thomas had arisen early every morning to make the family breakfast because of his mother's morning sickness.

By his own account, George was bashful and good natured, although, like his father, he could be violent when aroused. He noted that he was always "very fond of the fairer sex." When he was four, he walked half a mile to the farm of Louis La Rose and asked for the hand of his daughter, Minnie, in marriage. When asked by Louis what he possessed, he replied that he had a ten-acre field of his own, a colt, two pigs and a dog.

At first the one-room South Joliette school was open only in summer, but after three years it switched to the more usual winter schedule. George was needed in summer to help with chores since the Fergusons could not afford a hired man. By nine, he was driving a three-horse "sulky." George attended school for four winters, and when he was twelve he held his own in the Debating Society. That winter he contracted diphtheria and nearly died. He was left with chronic laryngitis and a husky voice which tended to make him even more bashful than usual.

A severe depression in the 1890s together with poor crops put many farmers, including Robert Ferguson, deeply in debt. The year he was fifteen George went back to school in January, February and March, after a three-year absence. An excellent teacher, E.P. Roe, taught him to work on his own. He had a good memory, liked history, geography, literature and mathematics, and passed his grade eight exams.

That year his nineteen-year-old brother, Jim, left to work in a store. By sixteen, George had taken Jim's place and was in full charge of the threshing crew "and the whole works," while his father looked after the farm and the hauling of grain. Father and son were great pals with never a difference between them. Indeed, George acted as the farm business manager. When a farm machinery salesman came to visit, Robert would ask his son whether the farm finances would allow the purchase of new equipment. George would get out the farm ledger, pore over it, make a few calculations, and usually say, "No father, they do not."

George was always "bookish." He borrowed from the neighbours and read everything he could get his hands on, even the textbooks his sisters brought home from school. He usually had a book in his pocket, even when on a gang plow. Already absent-minded, he would occasionally forget to do the chores. Until he was fifteen George was short and stout. Then he shot up to reach his final height of five feet eleven and a half inches at the age of seventeen. For the next twenty-five years he remained tall and thin.

Higher Education, 1902–1916

At the turn of the century the lure of free land drew people to Western Canada from all over the world. Many Americans sold their farms, put the proceeds in the bank, and moved north to begin over again on free land.

In 1902 nineteen-year-old George was sent by train from Winnipeg to Edmonton and Calgary, to seek a new homestead. Deciding that it was better to choose good land, some of it already broken, near a town, than to settle on a free homestead far from a railroad with no land under cultivation, George chose a farm at Yorkton, Saskatchewan, only one mile south of Broadway, the main street.

The east half of section 27, and the northeast quarter of section 22, township 25, range 4, west of the second meridian, 480 acres in total, describes the holding in a surveyor's terms. It was a large farm for the time, purchased by Robert Ferguson on 21 July 1902 from Yorkton merchant Levi Beck. Its proximity to the bustling town of Yorkton made this good land well worth the purchase price, said by the family to have been ten dollars an acre. The North Dakota farm of exactly the same size had been sold for twenty dollars an acre, which paid all Robert Ferguson's debts with some money left over. Ferguson took over an existing $2,500 mortgage at 9 percent annual interest and assumed an additional $2,000 mortgage payable to Levi Beck.[2] The north boundary of section 27 is now a paved bypass, joining Highways 9 and 10.

In October, George hired a team and plough from Jack Spice and worked until freeze-up, then became a boarder at the home of Mr. and Mrs. John Hawkins. Farmers paid part of their taxes by working on the roads with horses and a special type of grader blade known as a slush grader or frezenal. George graded a mile of road past the family farm towards York Lake. He was pleased when the mayor of Yorkton, impressed by the unusually straight road, asked him to "strike out" some of the Yorkton streets.

The next summer, when the family moved up from North Dakota (all but brother Jim and sister Eliza, and Ida May who had died of tuberculosis), George travelled eighty miles northwest, thinking he should take advantage of the availability of free land. On 29 June 1903 he filed on a homestead three miles north of Kuroki.[3] He failed to meet the homestead requirements (the breaking of ten acres and maintaining consecutive residence) imposed by government in exchange for the free grant of land, since he broke less than two acres that year. In his withdrawal deposition in Yorkton on 8 August 1905, George said he had found the property "too scrubby to be fit for profitable farming." The homestead was then purchased by a James Crawford, who built a house and barn, together valued at only $200, for his wife and three children. After five summers' work, Crawford was able to crop only sixteen-and-three-quarters acres, which bore out George's description of the land.

Inspired by E.P. Roe, his grade eight schoolteacher, George now determined to further his education. Accordingly, in 1904 he gained his father's permission to go to Wesley College in Winnipeg, to obtain grades nine and ten, junior matriculation (grade eleven) and senior matriculation (grade twelve), with a view to a career in the Methodist ministry.

On New Year's Day, 1906, when George was halfway through his Part II Matriculation, his father went to Bellingham, Washington, for treatment of pernicious anemia. Robert Ferguson was only fifty-five years old when he died there on 17 February 1906, twenty years before the discovery of liver extract as a remedy for this disease.

George was the oldest son in Canada, Jim having stayed behind in North Dakota. His mother, four younger brothers and six younger sisters lived on the farm. This quiet, serious young man, steeled by hard work and difficult times, now faced a tough decision. Should he take over operation of his father's farm? With his mother's strong encouragement and $600 left him by his father, George chose instead to complete his senior matriculation and then to embark on a three-year course in Arts.

All but two summers were spent back at the Yorkton farm, now owned by his mother, Margaret Jane Ferguson. The title deed registered her as "widow and administratrix of the estate," 30 September 1908, the property still carrying the original $2,500 mortgage. After three more additions the farm consisted in 1910 of seven quarter-sections or 1,120 acres, an unusually large farm for one so close to a growing town the size of Yorkton, but it was a time of unbridled optimism.[4] Unfortunately, the annual interest payments, most at 8 percent and 9 percent, proved to be a heavy burden.

In 1909 the Grand Trunk Pacific railway took 8.18 acres from the east half of section 27 as right-of-way for the Regina-Yorkton line. The Fergusons now had their own railway siding on the farm, and loaded their grain directly into boxcars parked at the siding.

Each year, as soon as he had written his last exam, George came home from Winnipeg to put in the crop to allow his brothers to continue their schooling. Each autumn, after taking off their own crop, George would move his threshing machine to one or more neighbouring farms. At noon, while the gang went off for dinner, George stayed in the field, oiling and greasing the machine, and adjusting the lacing to keep the belts tight. When the crew returned and the outfit was working smoothly again, one of his sisters would bring his dinner which always included an entire pie for dessert.

In the fall, the demands of farm work often meant that George returned late to his classes. One year it was the first of November before he could return to Winnipeg. His notebook for the academic year of 1907–08 shows that he received $167 from home and earned $72 from "Caskie," probably a neighbour for whom he harvested. After completing his second year in Arts, George spent the summer of 1908 in the Methodist mission field at Buchanan, Saskatchewan, where he cleared $139.45 for his summer's preaching, plus $25.80 in special offerings from parishioners and $5.00 from his mother. More important, he met Miss Helen Ross, who was visiting her brother Hervey, briefly in medical practice at Buchanan. In 1908–09 George won a scholarship of $100, and paid back a similar sum borrowed from his brother Tom. Although he was by now indebted to his mother for $464.65, she paid him $135 in wages for his summer's work in 1909.

George graduated Bachelor of Arts in 1910 and received the bronze medal, standing within one point of first in his class. He had been on the executive of the Wesley College Literary Society and his classmates elected him Senior Stick.

A classmate offered the following assessment of him in the Wesley College Yearbook:

> George Ferguson has got as much out of his college course as anyone . . . no finer a gentleman in its broadest sense ever graduated from Wesley College. From his father he inherited a deep sense of justice and honesty and from his mother patience

> and persistency. To this rich inheritance have been added as the years have gone by self-control, open-mindedness and sincerity . . . he has had . . . griefs and responsibilities to bear that would have crushed a less resolute heart. During the last four years of his college course he has been "the man of the house" and "the head of the family" . . . he has fulfilled the expectations and trust reposed in him, quiet, jovial, kind, always the same, he has won the respect of all and the love and esteem of many. No one appreciates his friends more and no one is more appreciated by his friends . . . he will always be found on the firing line and never sounding the retreat. Had George been more of an athlete he would have come as near the ideal college man as one could expect.

After a year of study in economics at the University of Manitoba, George put in a full year of Methodist mission work at Nobleford, Alberta. Here he realized that his husky voice did not have the strength and staying power to preach three sermons each Sunday. Years later he said that he never did know how well his sermons were appreciated by the congregation, but he knew that he gained the confidence of a parishioner each time he was able to repair or set the knotter on a binder. Since his voice was not adequate for the ministry, he chose the next best profession for serving humanity. He enrolled in the Manitoba College of Medicine in 1912. His notebook listed additional indebtedness of $175 to the Ferguson estate for his first year of medical studies.

Meanwhile, George's mother continued her role as farm manager. In 1912, according to Alec Engel, who now occupies the farm, she had a large nine-bedroom house constructed. Alec's uncle, Carl Engel, then aged seventeen, came in from Stornoway to haul the stones to build the barns. A horse barn, thirty-six feet by seventy-two feet, and a cattle barn, thirty feet by forty-eight feet, were built that summer by a German stonemason, with a well and windmill halfway between them. Each barn had a cement floor with gutters. These solidly constructed buildings are still standing. The house was built with beautiful hardwood floors, but it was cold, draughty and difficult to heat; it was torn down in 1946, the year after Fred Fiege purchased the farm.

By 5 January 1915 George's indebtedness to the estate had reached $618.50. In 1915–16 his college fees were $185, but he had earned $100 at

Ninette Sanatorium in the summer, after which he was paid $112.50 for one and a half month's work at the Winnipeg General Hospital. By 12 February 1916 he owed the estate $908.

In his final year George obtained needed extra money by working in the laboratory that made typhoid vaccine for the Canadian Army. He went to lectures in the morning, worked in the laboratory in the afternoon, slept from 6 p.m. till midnight and then studied until the university day began again. Dr. Harvey Boughton, whose room in the intern's quarters was across from his, reported that it was easiest for George to study when others were asleep. Because of this unusual schedule, his classmates saw very little of him.

The University of Manitoba Class and Honour Lists for 1916 show that, in spite of his heavy extracurricular load, George placed second in his class in the final year of medicine. First place went to William Frederick Abbott, a surgeon who founded the Abbott Clinic in Winnipeg. Abbott had straight 1As, equivalent to A-plus. George received this top grade in clinical medicine, clinical surgery, operative surgery, and "ophthalmology, etc.," and the grade of 1B, equivalent to A-minus, in theoretical medicine, theoretical surgery, and obstetrics. Clearly he was good in his theoretical subjects but even better in their practical application on the wards.

Following graduation in 1916 George made a brief trip east to write, and pass, the Dominion Council examinations. He became Licentiate #300 of the Medical Council of Canada, and thereby qualified to practise in any province.

On 5 July 1916, after a four-year engagement, George married his sweetheart of eight years. He listed his marriage expenses at $100. His twenty-four-year-old bride, Helen Ross, was the daughter of Thomas Hervey Ross, an insurance salesman, and the granddaughter of Dr. Hervey Thomas Ross of Burford, Ontario. Helen's mother, Maria Augusta Elliott, was the daughter of Daniel Elliott and Maria Smith of Burford, Ontario. The Ross family had moved to Wynyard, Saskatchewan, in 1911. Helen, the only girl, had four living brothers: Heber Huillet Ross, a veterinary surgeon who remained at Burford; Carman, who worked in the Wynyard drug store and died of influenza in 1918; Hervey Reginald Ross, who registered with the Saskatchewan College of Physicians and Surgeons, on 18 November 1909; Gordon Winniford Ross, who registered on 23 January 1911. The two medical brothers together owned and operated a hospital in Wynyard for two years, but sold their practice and moved to Assiniboia, Saskatchewan, in 1913, and later to British Columbia. The fifth brother, Hervey Alfonso ("Alley"), had died early in life.

Helen had studied Art at Moulton College, Toronto, before moving to Wynyard. In 1913, less than a year after becoming engaged to George Ferguson, she entered training at the Winnipeg General Hospital. She contracted scarlet fever, diphtheria and pneumonia near the end of her third year and was unable to complete her nursing training.

In the summer of 1916 George began work under Dr. A.B. Alexander as assistant superintendent of the municipal hospitals in Winnipeg, taking over from Dr. A.T. Mathers, who later became a psychiatrist and dean of medicine at the University of Manitoba. The newlyweds were very happy. Each had classmates working in Winnipeg hospitals, and their social life revolved around them. A son, Robert, was born on 13 May 1917. At the end of June they moved to Fort Qu'Appelle, Saskatchewan, to undertake a new challenge.

— Chapter Two —

Founding of the Anti-tuberculosis League

"The captain of these men of death that came against him to take him away, was the Consumption, for it was that that brought him down to the grave."
John Bunyan, 1628–1688, *The Life and Death of Mr. Badman*

THE INITIAL IMPETUS for the anti-tuberculosis program in Saskatchewan was provided by Dr. Maurice M. Seymour, then provincial health commissioner and later the deputy minister of public health. His work in Saskatchewan was internationally known, serving as a model for other provinces and countries, notably the "Seymour Plan" for combatting typhoid, diphtheria and smallpox. But his anti-tuberculosis project suffered many frustrations before Dr. R.G. Ferguson arrived to give leadership and direction.

In 1907, Dr. Seymour's son had developed tuberculosis and was taken to the tuberculosis sanatorium of Dr. Edward Livingstone Trudeau at Saranac Lake, New York. Seymour learned from Trudeau that tuberculosis could be arrested. That year he recommended to Premier Walter Scott and his government that "provision be made at once for the establishment of a sanatorium which will afford a means of cure for early cases, and what is, I think, of very great importance, a means of isolating the advanced and incurable cases in a way that will prevent them being a cause of communicating the disease to others."

In the meantime, Seymour advocated isolation wards in existing general hospitals and increased education of the public. Not until early 1911 was Seymour able to obtain the services of Dr. George D. Porter of

Ottawa, who had been appointed in 1908 as the first full-time secretary of the Canadian Tuberculosis Association. Seymour then called a general meeting in the King's Hotel, Regina, on 17 February 1911, for the purpose of "organizing a Provincial Anti-tuberculosis League and interviewing the Government with reference to a grant for a sanatorium for early cases, and a hospital for advanced cases of tuberculosis." Peter McAra, the mayor of Regina, was elected president and Dr. Seymour, secretary. Others present were James Campbell, B.B. Carter, John McCarthy, Thomas Molloy, and Dr. E.E. Meek, all from Regina; Canon Frederick Wells Johnson and Dr. Robert Gibson from Moose Jaw; John R. Bunn, M. Isbister, and Dr. W.J. McKay of Saskatoon; A. Davidson and Dr. F.W. Hart from Indian Head; R.S. Moore of Swift Current; John Dixon of Maple Creek; H.A. Hastings of Rouleau; and Dr. William Sinclair of Manor.

These men of action allowed no grass to grow under their feet; they drove that very day to the parliament buildings where they had an audience with the three key members of the provincial cabinet: the Honourable Walter Scott, premier; the Honourable J.A. Calder, provincial treasurer and minister of education, railways, telegraphs and telephones; and the Honourable William Richard Motherwell, provincial secretary and minister of agriculture. Seymour, McAra, Wells Johnson, Bunn, Isbister, Dixon, Dr. Hart and the two health officers present, Drs. Meek and McKay, all addressed the politicians. Premier Scott "expressed sympathy with the movement and promised that the Government would give the matter its most earnest consideration."

The delegation went back to the hotel and elected M. Isbister as first vice-president, John Dixon as second vice-president, J.H. Francis of Indian Head as third vice-president, and B.B. Carter as treasurer. For their honorary positions they chose carefully: Lieutenant Governor G.W. Brown as honorary president and Premier Scott and F.W.G. Haultain, leader of the opposition, as the two honorary vice-presidents.

For nearly two months, Seymour and Porter carried the message to Saskatchewan communities. They had a standard plan. Insofar as possible, a meeting was scheduled in each of the forty-one electoral divisions in the province. Posters were placed in advance. Usually the mayor or a local medical doctor was asked to preside over the public meeting. No admission was charged. A yearly membership fee of one dollar per person was established, seventy-five cents of this going to the provincial headquarters.

The first meeting outside Regina was held on 21 February 1911 at Lloydminster. Porter was eloquent, urging the need for prevention and for fresh-air treatment. Everyone was advised to sleep with a window open. Seymour was optimistic, hoping to establish a province-wide league and to begin construction within the year of the first sanatorium building, estimated to cost $50,000. The government was expected to match the money donated and pay for the second building.

Meetings at Carnduff, Estevan, Weyburn, Whitewood, Wapella, Davidson, Moose Jaw, Indian Head, Saskatoon, Wolseley, Prince Albert, Davidson, Grenfell, Regina, Lumsden and Moosomin were held between 10 March and 16 May. The turnout at many points was disappointing, yet those present were asked to form a local branch of the Anti-tuberculosis League and elect officers. At Weyburn, the enthusiastic new committee collected nearly $400 from local businessmen the very next day.

The League directors were first-rate in their ability to make contacts with politicians but were less successful as money-raisers. Incorporation of the Saskatchewan Anti-tuberculosis League (henceforth simply called the League) became Chapter 10 of the legislation passed on 23 March 1911 during the 1910–11 session of the provincial legislature – before the public meetings had even been completed! Supplementary estimates of $25,000 had also been included, to be given the League when it had collected $25,000 from the public.

The 1911 annual meeting of the Canadian Association for the Prevention of Tuberculosis listed active branches of the League at Abernethy, Battleford, Carnduff, Davidson, Estevan, Fleming, Grenfell, Hanley, Indian Head, Lumsden, Milestone, Moose Jaw, Moosomin, Prince Albert, Regina, Saskatoon, Wapella, Weyburn, Whitewood and Wolseley. These were in the cities and the more established communities east of Regina and between Regina and Saskatoon.

At their meeting of 13 June 1911 the League directors agreed to appoint Dr. William Malloch Hart of Duluth, Minnesota, as medical superintendent at $4,000 per year and a house once the sanatorium was built. Hart had been a patient at the Trudeau Sanatorium in 1907 when Seymour first met him. Born in Winnipeg, he had obtained B.A. and M.D. degrees from the University of Manitoba, graduating in 1907.

Hart began his official duties on 1 September 1911. Dr. Seymour met Hart in Winnipeg and together they visited the Manitoba Sanatorium at Ninette. "Among other things we learned during our visit, that most important . . . in the selection of a site for a sanatorium is accessibility to the larger centres of population. Manitoba has made a serious mistake in this respect, as it takes two long days from Winnipeg to visit the Sanatorium at Ninette."

The three-man committee appointed in April 1911 to select a site for the sanatorium buildings consisted of M. Isbister of Saskatoon (later replaced by Dr. Seymour), Dr. Frederick William Hart of Indian Head (no relation to the first medical superintendent, Dr. William Malloch Hart) and Mr. John Dixon of Maple Creek. Initially there had been enthusiasm for a site in the wooded portion of the Cypress Hills in extreme southwestern Saskatchewan, where 60,000 acres had recently been set aside by the Dominion government for forest preservation. A ranch had been planned in association with the sanatorium to allow the patients to do outdoor work. The committee, however, found the theory of outdoor manual labour somewhat discredited by this time and for the convenience of patients and family chose a more central site. As a result of its report in March 1912, a parcel of 230 acres on the north shore of Echo Lake, west of Fort Qu'Appelle, was purchased by the directors of the League for $8,250. This sum was partially offset by a donation of $3,000 from the municipality of North Qu'Appelle and the village of Fort Qu'Appelle. Other encouraging news came from the provincial government; it offered to increase its support to $60,000, payable if and when the League could raise another $40,000 from public subscriptions.

The chosen site, an attractive semi-circular haven facing the sun and ensconced within a series of hills protecting it from north winds, even had the support of John Dixon, who was from the bypassed southwest corner of the province. Architect J.H. Puntin prepared detailed plans for buildings worth $93,000, while Joseph Campbell took over as president of the League.

Seymour had been a general practitioner at Lebret. His old stone house on the north side of the lake, almost halfway between Lebret and Fort Qu'Appelle, was later donated to the Boy Scouts of Canada. He loved the valley and for the rest of his life took great pride in his part in having helped choose the site of the Fort Qu'Appelle Sanatorium; he maintained his personal interest in the institution, dropping in to visit on every possible occasion.

In the same year Miss Mabel Scott, a graduate nurse, was hired for $100 per month to organize fund-raising tag days which had generated

$30,000 revenue in Manitoba the year before. She was sent to Winnipeg to see how its campaign had been organized. She purchased 75,000 "medals" at 2.5 cents each to give to each donor. Mrs. McKaugh was hired to help Miss Scott. The first tag days were an enormous amount of work, with proceeds of $20,295 and expenses of $6,580.40. The 1913 tag day was a disaster and cleared only $604.75. The "worthless medallions," carried on the books with a value of $1,331.25, were finally written off by the League in January 1918.

A full-time executive secretary, Arthur T. Samuel, was added to the staff in September 1912, at a salary of $2,500 per year. Miss Riddell was the stenographer.

In the fall of 1912, George R. Milan, an experienced fund-raiser from the Trudeau Sanatorium, was engaged at $125 per month on three months' probation; he was replaced by George Dean on 10 January 1913, but Dean resigned on 15 April and R.H. Bothwell was then appointed canvasser at $100 per month with $25 allowance for use of his car. Dr. W.M. Hart himself took care of canvassing in Regina, as he had no patients to care for – but fund-raising was not one of his talents. He found it hard going owing to the tightness of the money market and the season of the year. The directors had asked Dr. Hart to interview every minister in Regina, and "arrange for sermons to be given on tuberculosis in their churches next Sunday if possible."

Seymour's initial optimism for a sanatorium opening in 1912 proved unrealistic. The League's fund-raising drive sputtered along in an inept manner, garnering a lot of promises but very little hard cash. The canvassers in 1912 collected only $520, but obtained promissory notes which by February 1913, totalled $25,468, some of them not due until 1917, in addition to the $9,530 in promissory notes already due but not paid. On the CPR main line east, donations averaged just under thirty-three cents each, which hardly paid the salary and expenses of the canvasser. Money collected in the first three years was little more than enough to purchase the site and pay for the expenses of the full-time League staff and fund-raisers. A depression set in and many donors were unable to honour their promissory notes. Worse, the League had no buildings to show for the donations received.

In May 1913 the League called for tenders for the administration building, two pavilions, and the superintendent's residence. The lowest tender came in at $118,000 without the power house, water storage or sewer disposal. The contract was awarded to Parsons Construction in

July 1913, but construction was stalled for lack of funds. At the end of 1913 the League gained a forceful new president, Regina Sheriff A.B. Cook, but it had only $1,526.28 in hand.

Construction finally got under way in the early summer of 1914, only to be halted by the trustees meeting of 4 July, when minutes record that they had now reached the limit of their financial resources with no expectation of being able to resume building during either 1914 or 1915. To continue construction, the League was able to negotiate a $95,000 loan from the government to be repaid in eight equal annual instalments with interest – an impossible task in view of the League's poor track record in raising money by voluntary donations. The offer became known on 3 August, the day before war was declared.

Dr. W.M. Hart immediately enlisted, leaving the League on 15 August. His patriotism had a tangible benefit to himself – he could thus escape from what must have seemed an untenable situation of boredom and imminent failure. For nearly three years he had been the administrator of a limping organization which provided him little satisfaction and rarely used any of his medical skills. On arrival in England, Hart was appointed medical officer of the Fifth Battalion.

The League, too, had an honourable escape from commitments which it could not meet. Its funds were exhausted. The outlook for further assistance from the government was bleak. Men and materials were needed for the war effort. Construction at Fort Qu'Appelle came to a standstill and the buildings, valued at $94,932.82, were boarded up. In 1915, the YMCA was allowed to use one of the buildings as sleeping accommodation for the boys at their summer camp, and in November a watchman was engaged at $50 per month.

Things began to look up in November 1915 when the Military Hospitals Commission of Canada enquired what part of the sanatorium was now in readiness and how many servicemen might be accommodated. The needs of sick soldiers spurred the League in April 1916 to complete the superintendent's residence and one pavilion. In August 1917 Sheriff Cook came back from a year of overseas service. As the Dominion government invalided home with tuberculosis increasing numbers of Canadian soldiers, Judge Edward Lindsay Elwood, official representative of the Military Hospitals Commission, attended the League directors' meeting of 19 February 1917. The Dominion government advanced $150,000 to complete an infirmary and two cottages, and to purchase furnishings for the buildings already constructed.

The war, which had provided an excuse to cease building in 1914, now became the salvation of the sanatorium. Federal money allowed preparations for occupancy of the sanatorium to proceed at full speed. But it was Dr. Ferguson's arrival on 1 July 1917 as acting superintendent that planted the Saskatchewan anti-tuberculosis program on the road to success as the first grassroots, one-disease organization in Saskatchewan.

Ferguson's Mentor, Dr. David A. Stewart

Dr. David A. Stewart was Dr. Ferguson's mentor and exemplar. Stewart's pioneer and innovative program for training medical students at the Ninette Sanatorium became compulsory for all University of Manitoba medical students in 1914 and continued through the 1950s. Stewart had recognized young Ferguson's potential when he was a medical student working for his summer board and lodging at the Ninette Sanatorium. Ferguson accepted responsibility so well that Stewart turned to him when he needed someone to run the sanatorium to allow him time for his already delayed wedding and honeymoon in June 1915. Both of his assistants, Dr. C.A. Baragar and Dr. Baldur Olson, had left for war service. The trustworthy medical student, Robert George Ferguson, looked after all administrative matters for the month, while Dr. Harvey Boughton came to care for the patients.

Two years later, with Dr. W.M. Hart on wartime service and the new sanatorium about to open, Sheriff A.B. Cook, the president of the Saskatchewan Anti-tuberculosis League, phoned Stewart. Did he know anyone who could serve as acting medical director? Without hesitation, Stewart recommended Ferguson. If, when only a medical student, he could run Ninette, he was the man Saskatchewan needed.

Stewart, on excellent terms with the Manitoba Association of Rural Municipalities, each year attended its annual meeting to report on progress at the Ninette Sanatorium. Ferguson and Cook, anxious to gain the confidence of the Saskatchewan Association of Rural Municipalities (SARM) in a similar way, decided it would be best if the more experienced Stewart were to "break the ice." Stewart was given a splendid hearing as guest speaker at the SARM annual meeting at Moose Jaw on 6 March 1918. He reported to Ferguson that the municipalities would likely provide considerable financial help to the sanatorium, as indeed they did.

Stewart and Ferguson kept in close touch throughout their careers, sharing ideas and programs. On their visits, which alternated between Ninette and Fort Qu'Appelle, they often brought with them other members of their family and staff.

David Alexander Stewart, born on 15 February 1874, in Fletcher, Kent County, Ontario, was the son of Francis Beattie Stewart and Elizabeth Farquharson Stewart, and the nephew of James Farquharson, the home mission superintendent of the Presbyterian Church for Manitoba and the Northwest Territories. His father, although a farmer and not ordained, came west to serve at mission stations in rural Manitoba in 1891. After attending Normal School (teacher training school) in Winnipeg in 1893, David taught at Clegg near Morden until he entered the Faculty of Arts at Manitoba College in 1896. He then studied theology for two years, planning to become a Presbyterian minister.

In 1902, David's last summer posting as a student missionary was at Frank, Alberta. There he became friendly with Dr. George H. Malcolmson, who ran a small hospital beside his house. Malcolmson's influence apparently motivated David to abandon theology, to his father's great disappointment, and enter the Manitoba Medical College in the fall of 1902. Just as his first-year examinations ended, he heard of the devastating landslide from the top of Turtle Mountain which covered most of the little mining town of Frank on 29 April 1903. Because of his familiarity with the town, the *Manitoba Free Press* agreed to pay his way to Frank in return for daily reports. Stewart worked all summer alongside Dr. Malcolmson, whose only nurse had taken fright and fled. The doctor's assistant and nurse by day, he wrote his *Free Press* reports by night. Early each morning he climbed the mountain to measure the cracks which had formed behind the peak, to look for evidence of any further rock movement.

Thus began Stewart's job as a part-time reporter with the *Free Press*, which paid his way through medical school and put him under the tutelage of the dean of Canadian newspapermen, John Wesley Dafoe. Stewart obtained his M.D. in 1906. As a senior intern, the first to hold this position at the Winnipeg General Hospital, he continued occasional assignments for the newspaper, including an interview with Dr. Robert Koch, the discoverer of the tubercle bacillus, when Koch passed through Winnipeg on 14 September 1908.

That year Stewart was named by the new Manitoba Sanatorium Board as their first executive officer whose responsibilities included teaching the public about tuberculosis and the raising of funds for a sanatorium. Travelling widely across the province and working hard with an irregular schedule, he succumbed to the very disease he was seeking to heal in others. Stewart went for treatment at the famous Trudeau Sanatorium at Saranac Lake, New York.

Meanwhile, in his absence the new sanatorium at Ninette opened on 20 May 1910. It was the first sanatorium in a Prairie province. Stewart returned to work full-time in November, and had no recurrence of tuberculosis.

Saskatchewan followed the Ninette example. Stewart and Ferguson faced almost identical problems: the overwhelming influx of servicemen towards the last half of the war (which resulted in the injection of federal funds to build three large pavilions at Ninette), the incredibly high rates of tuberculosis among the Indians (in Manitoba, 30 to 45 percent of tuberculosis victims were Indian, although Indians formed only 2 percent of the total population), the perennial shortage of funds and the need to get the most out of every dollar (Ninette operated at Canada's lowest cost per patient day). Sometimes it was Stewart, sometimes Ferguson, who first began a program. Travelling clinics began in Saskatchewan in 1924 and in Manitoba in 1926; Christmas Seal funding began in Manitoba in 1927 and in Saskatchewan in 1928.

In 1915, David Stewart married Ida Kate Bradshaw, a registered nurse; she was thirty-seven and he was forty-two. She had a strong social conscience and was a great inspiration to her husband. After David Bradshaw Stewart was born on 18 June 1916, she contracted pulmonary tuberculosis. When Ida did not improve with rest and treatment, first at Ninette and then at Gravenhurst Sanatorium in Ontario, she underwent thoracoplasty in 1925 at the hands of Dr. Edward Archibald of Montreal. Although considerably improved and no longer infectious, she remained a semi-invalid and died in 1936.

In spite of increasingly debilitating chronic illness, diverticulitis of the colon with chronic pelvic abscess, Stewart continued writing about tuberculosis, philosophy, and Western Canadian history until his death in 1937. His talents in the literary, philosophic and religious fields made him the ideal person to draft the first Code of Ethics adopted by the Canadian Medical Association. His eight articles, "Things of the Spirit: The Sick Man's Religion," initially published in the *Journal of the Outdoor Life*, the educational journal for tuberculosis patients initiated by the Trudeau Sanatorium, were widely acclaimed and frequently reprinted.

In many ways Ferguson and Stewart followed a similar path. Both were men of vision, with a clear purpose. Though neither gave a high priority to formal religion, each retained a missionary zeal, studying the Bible and living an exemplary life.

As intellectuals, they shared an interest in Indians and the history of exploration of Western Canada; they were members of the Champlain Society. Ferguson's paper on tuberculosis among Cree Indians was a highlight of the National Association for the Prevention of Tuberculosis in London, England, in 1928, and Stewart's paper on the explorer Dr. John Richardson, surgeon and naturalist with the first two arctic exploring expeditions led by John Franklin, was an equally memorable event at the combined meeting of the British and Canadian Medical Associations in Winnipeg in 1930.

Each was a prolific writer, teacher, and evangelist of the prevention/education message. Stewart wrote: "Teachers must not only possess truth; they must be possessed by it . . . Teaching is the thing. The body that has been healed, at the very best cannot last forever, but must sooner or later be swept away by the ruthless on-rush of time. Teaching is more permanent than healing. Ideas live." In a day when few medical doctors in Western Canada contributed to the medical literature, each wrote important papers and encouraged their staff in research projects. Stewart's bibliography lists fifty-nine papers and Ferguson's, twenty-two.

Both were highly respected by the medical community. Stewart was elected president of the Manitoba Medical Association in 1926, four years after Ferguson was president of the Saskatchewan Medical Association. The University of Manitoba granted Stewart an honorary LL.D. in 1927 and the University of Saskatchewan gave Ferguson one in 1946. Stewart was also president of the Manitoba Historical and Scientific Society from 1929 through 1934.

Above all, they were idealists who harnessed almost unlimited energy to their cause. They followed the dictum of St. Benedict: "The care of the sick is to be placed above and before every other duty, as if, indeed, Christ were being directly served in waiting on them."

When Stewart died, after a lingering illness, on 16 February 1937, it was Ferguson who wrote his memorial in the *Journal of Thoracic Surgery*. And it was Ferguson who described himself as Stewart's disciple when he gave the annual David A. Stewart Memorial Lecture at the University of Manitoba in 1942.

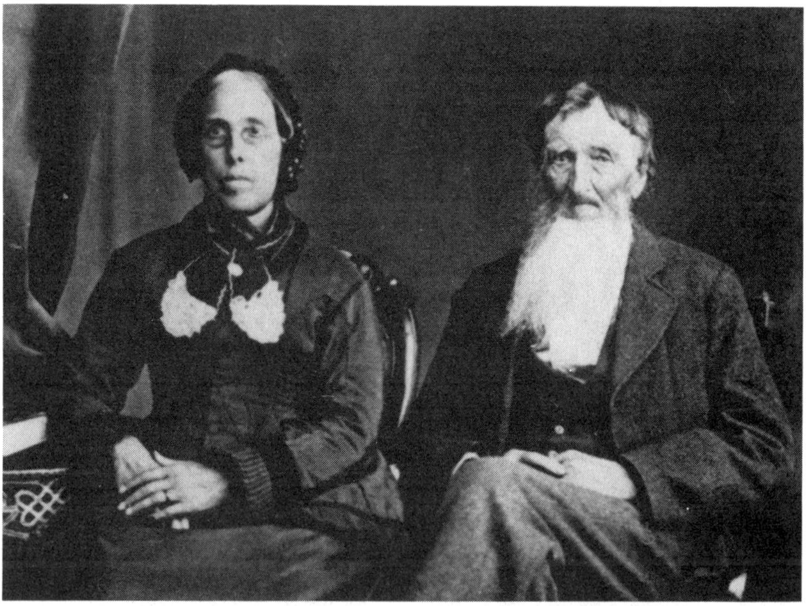

Courtesy of the Ferguson family

James Ferguson (1814–1902) and third wife, Frances Jordan Ferguson.

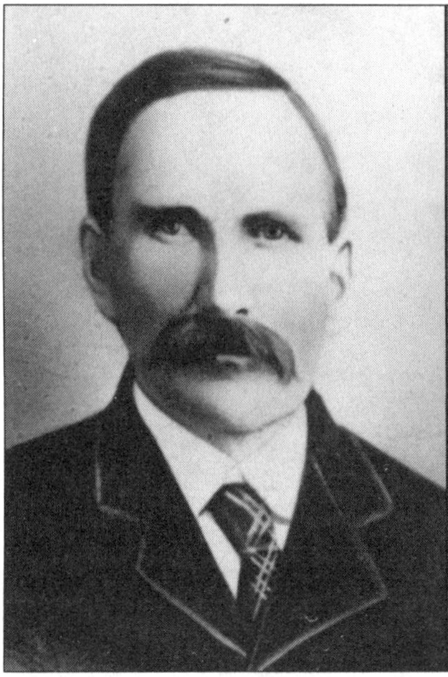

Courtesy of the Ferguson family

Robert Ferguson
(16 August 1850 – 17 February 1906).

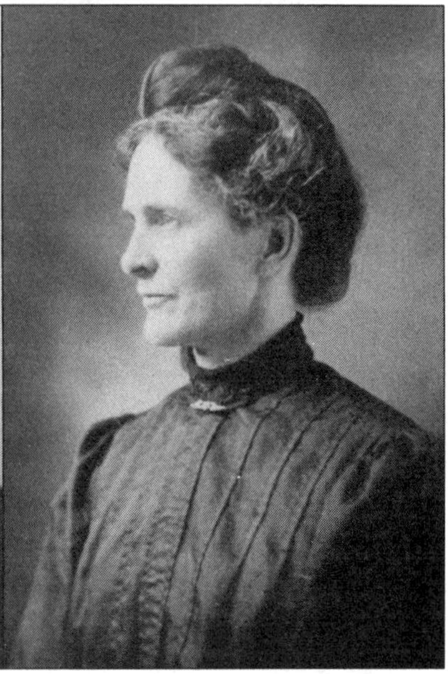

Courtesy of the Ferguson family

Margaret Jane (Fisher) Ferguson
(7 June 1855 – 21 January 1948).

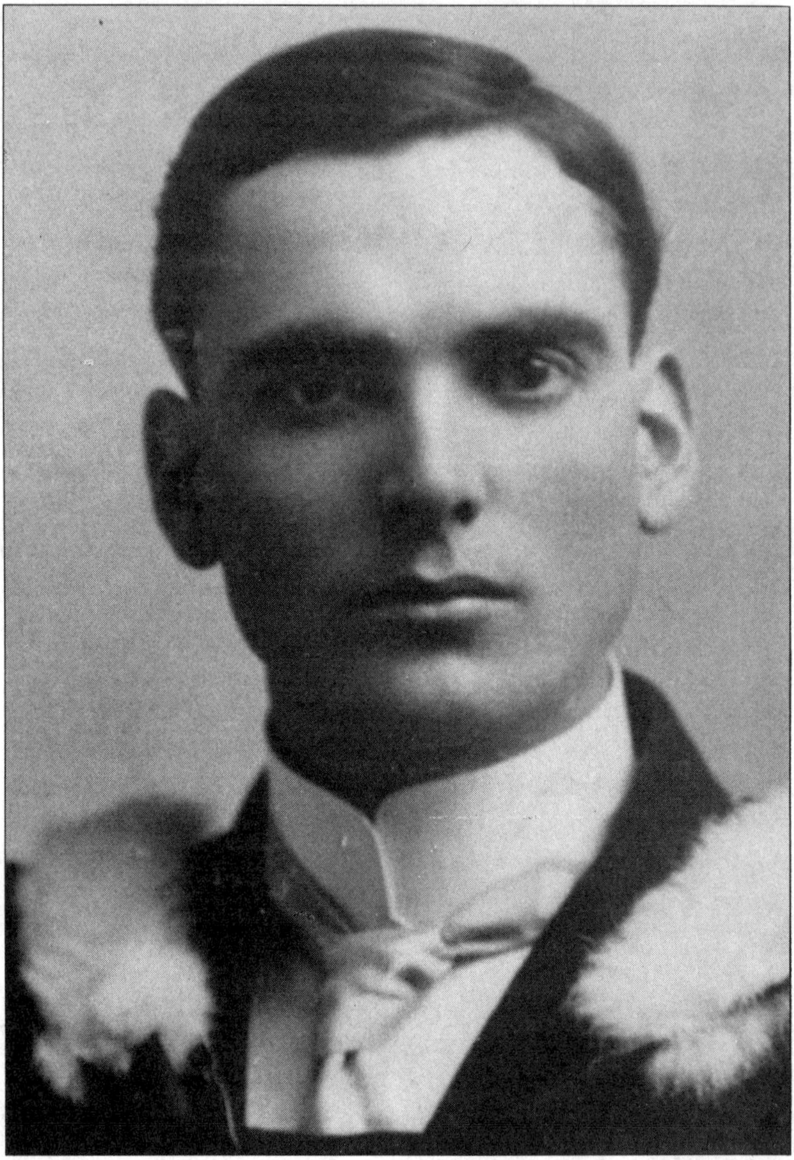

Courtesy of the Saskatchewan Lung Association

R.G. Ferguson, M.D., May 1916.

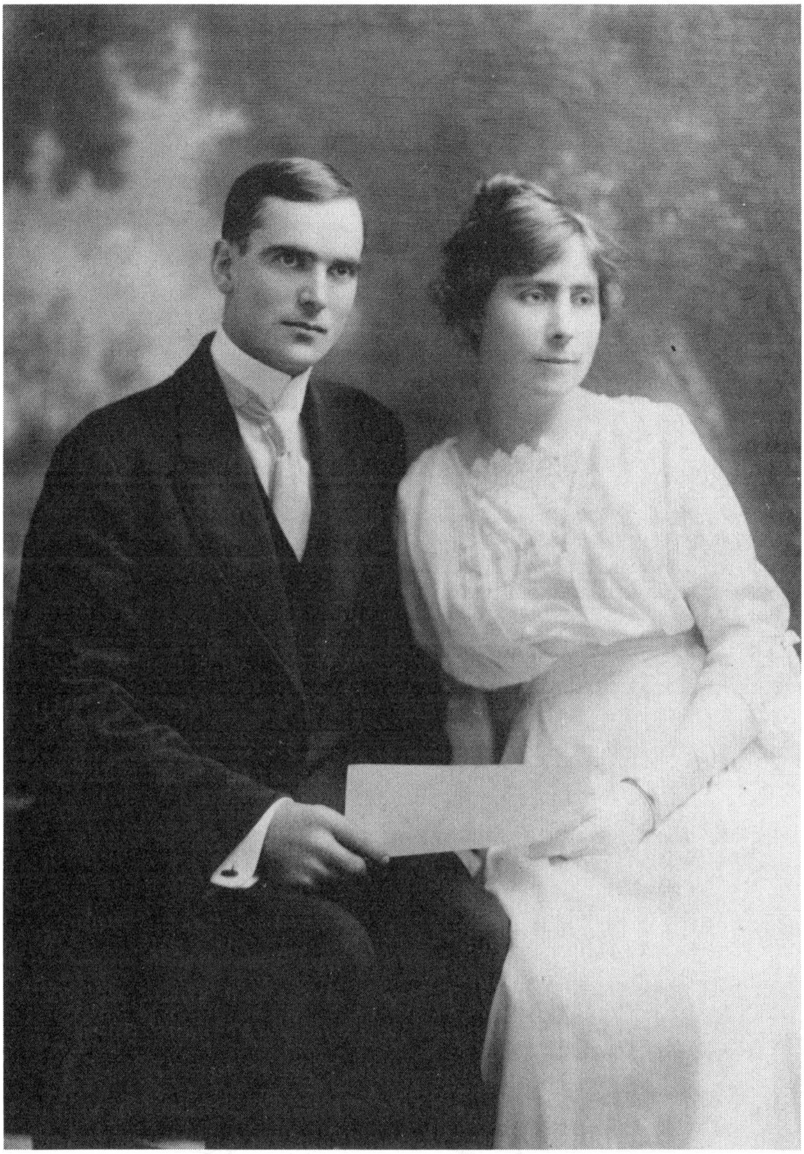

Courtesy of the Saskatchewan Lung Association

George and Helen (Ross) Ferguson, wedding photo, 5 July 1916.

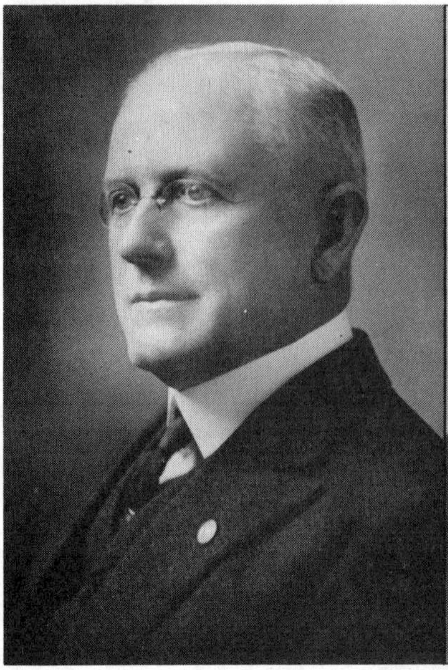

Courtesy of the Ferguson family

Dr. Maurice Macdonald Seymour
(7 July 1857 – 17 January 1929).

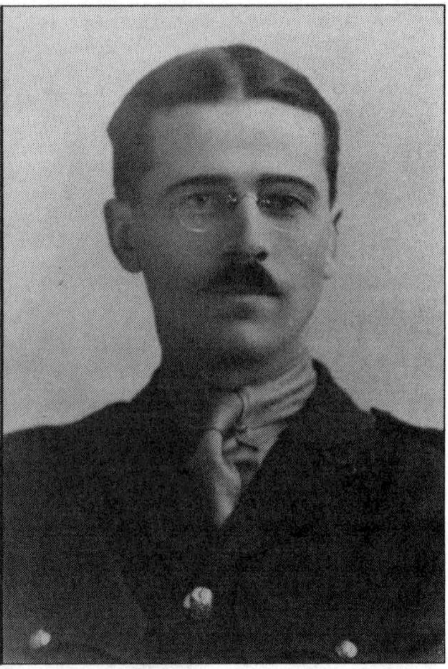

Courtesy of the Saskatchewan Lung Association

Dr. William Malloch Hart
(d. 1923).

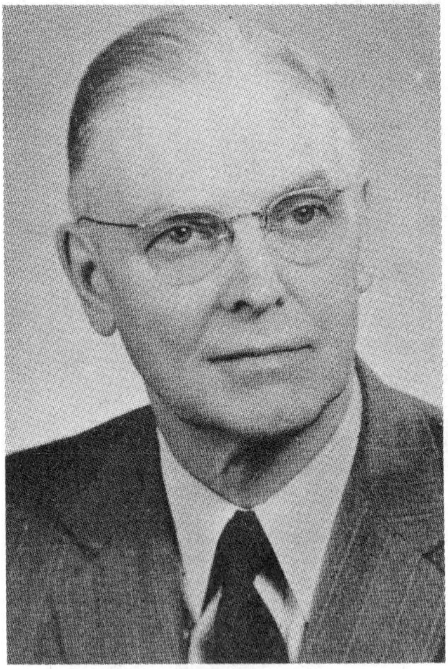

Courtesy of the Saskatchewan Lung Association

Dr. Harvey Crawford Boughton
(16 April 1889 – 26 May 1970).

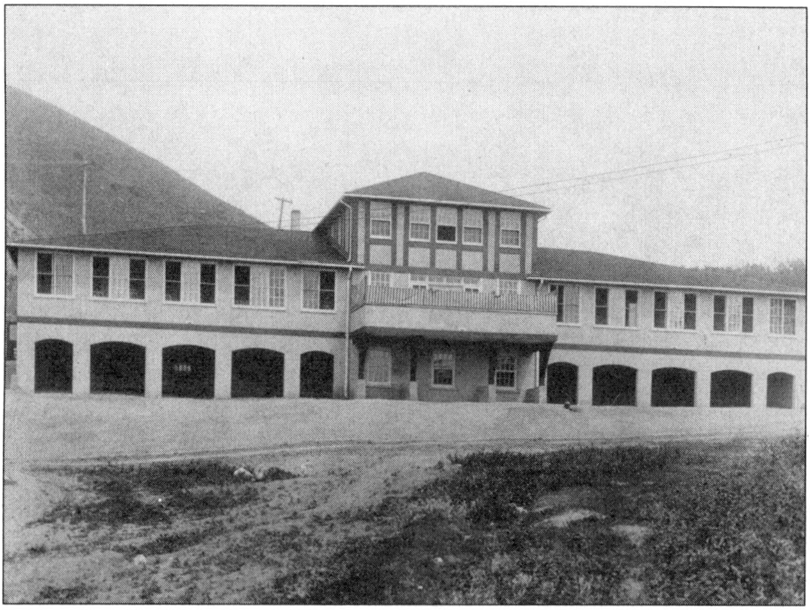

Courtesy of Henry Daneleyko

Children's Pavilion, Fort San, 1919.

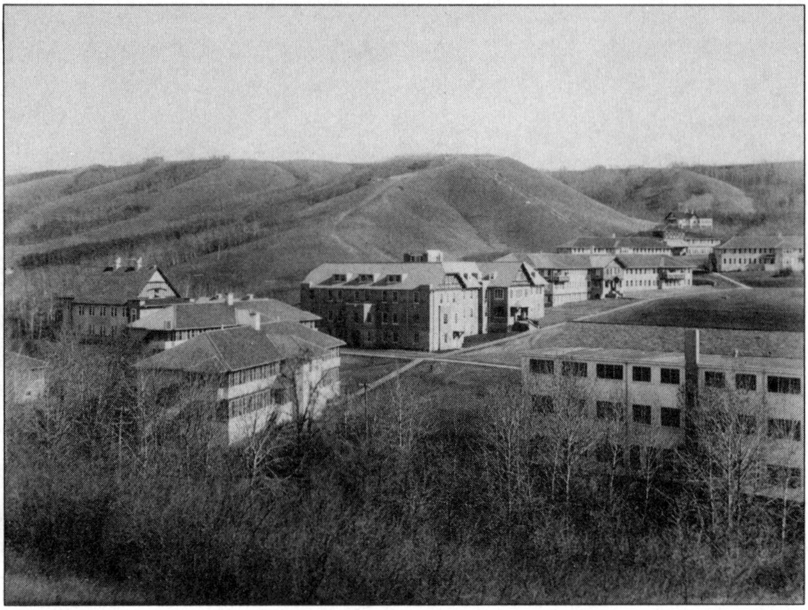

Courtesy of the Ferguson family

Fort San, ca. 1922.

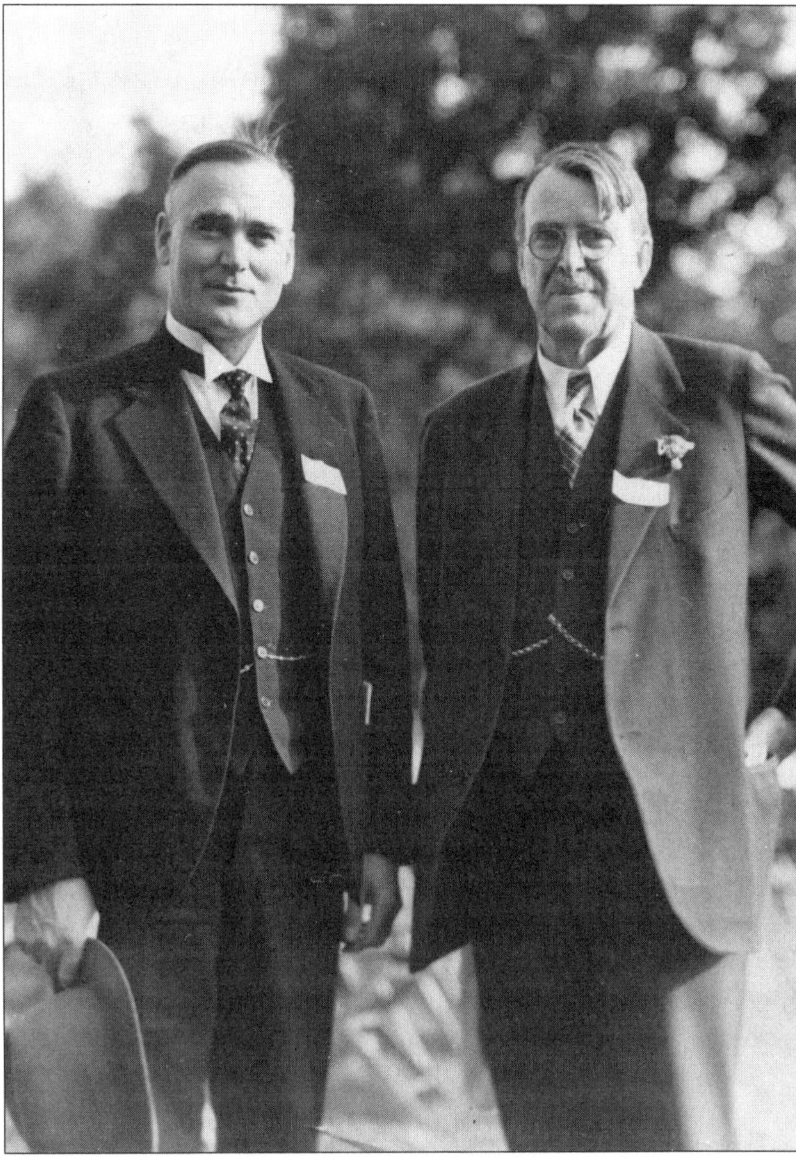

Courtesy of Henry Daneleyko

R.G. Ferguson and David A. Stewart (15 February 1874 – 16 February 1937) in 1935.

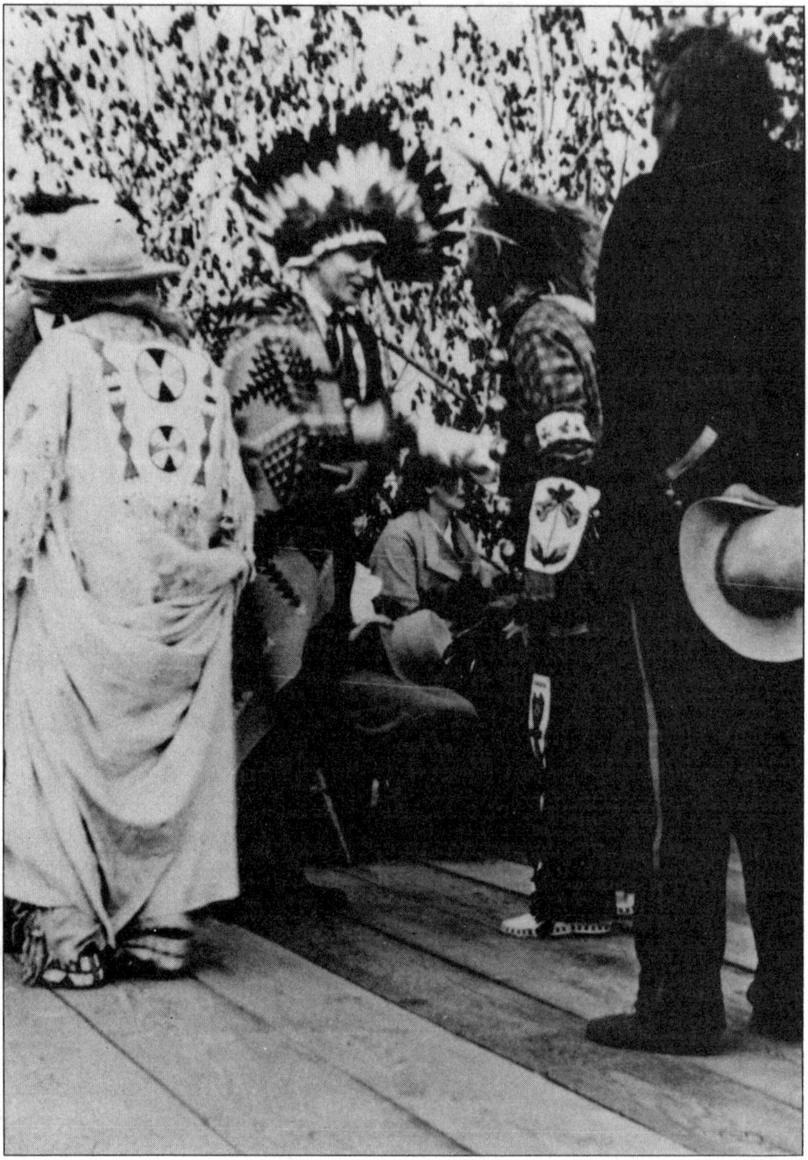

Courtesy of the Saskatchewan Lung Association

Chief Muskeke-O-Kemacan (Great White Physician), 24 May 1935.

— Chapter Three —
Fort San

Ferguson's Appointment, 1917

ON THE RECOMMENDATION of Dr. Stewart, the League asked Dr. Ferguson to come to Saskatchewan as its acting medical superintendent for six months pending the return of Dr. William Malloch Hart from overseas service.

At the first meeting of the League after his appointment in July, Ferguson offered to do without electric power in his new $10,000 residence on the hill for the first winter and to use coal oil lamps instead because of the heavy cost of stringing temporary copper wire from the power house to the residence. He also advised the directors to decline an offer by Parsons Construction Company of a team of horses and wagon, a driving horse, harness and buggy, one set of sleighs and one cutter for the sum of $600. Ferguson argued that the "team was too light for the heavy work of hauling coal and supplies to the Sanatorium . . . the driving horse too ancient, and the sleighs and cutter practically useless." The board appointed their vice-president, J.H. Francis of Indian Head, to serve with Ferguson as a special committee of two to purchase a team of horses, harness, cutter and sleighs. As it happened, Francis himself donated a "team of greys" and the harness a few months later.

Ferguson faced a pretty hopeless task. At that time there was a "close direct relation" between the general death rate and the tuberculosis death rate. Tuberculosis was widespread throughout Saskatchewan, with about 400 deaths yearly among the 700,000 inhabitants of the newly settled province. Another thousand "broke down" each year with the disease. The afflicted were typically at the prime of life with maximum responsibilities, yet the men found themselves unable to work and provide for their families and the women unable to care for their children. Indeed, tuberculosis was frequently passed from parent to child especially among new immigrants when a family was often crowded into a one-room shack.

The disease was difficult to diagnose because the symptoms were vague and non-specific. The chest radiograph was helpful but rather insensitive, especially since few doctors had yet learned to discern early lesions at the apex of the lung. The tuberculin skin test was not always reliable. By the time the sputum was positive, the disease was far advanced and highly contagious.

Often five years elapsed between infection and breakdown. Many patients had had tuberculosis for years, some already "open" and contagious, before they realized they were ill. This long lag made it a difficult disease to conquer. The only good news was that since Robert Koch's identification of the tuberculosis bacillus in 1882, the disease was at least known not to be hereditary.

In Saskatchewan, particularly, general hospitals could not be part of the solution. They were too small and too widely scattered. At the turn of the century Saskatchewan had only three hospitals, the Grey Nuns Hospital in the far north at Île-à-la-Crosse, the Regina Cottage Hospital and the Prince Albert Hospital, each with seven beds. Another thirty hospitals were in operation by World War I, but few beds could be spared for long-term treatment of tuberculosis. Even if beds had been available, most patients could not afford to stay for the many months or years required for adequate treatment and isolation. And most physicians and nurses lacked the knowledge and training necessary for optimal care of the disease.

A few well-off family members who developed tuberculosis were sent to the Trudeau Sanatorium in Saranac, New York. Facilities there were extremely limited — at its peak it could accommodate only 125 patients in twenty-five cottages. But even the renowned Trudeau

Sanatorium had little to offer except rest, fresh air, sunlight and good food. There was as yet no proven method of vaccination against tuberculosis. Injections of tuberculin, the protein produced by tubercle bacilli in culture, popularized by Koch as a treatment, had proved ineffective.

No wonder the medical profession and governments were perplexed. In most parts of the world uncertainty led to apathy and inaction. Many governments were unwilling to put much time or effort or money into fighting tuberculosis, since the majority of sanatorium patients in England, in spite of treatment, died of tuberculosis within a few years. The public had not yet developed faith in institutionalized medicine.

Saskatchewan, a new province, with new settlers who hadn't really found their feet, was a most improbable place for programs destined to lead North America. Yet Ferguson led his chosen province to embark on a visionary if expensive course, building more sanatoria beds per tuberculosis patient and more beds per tuberculosis death than any other jurisdiction.[1] High capital costs combined with high costs of identifying patients with the disease, while good results were by no means guaranteed.

Why was impoverished Saskatchewan a leader? The answer relates, in part, to the calibre of the man chosen to direct its program, Robert George Ferguson, and the strong support his own conviction generated. Where else could Ferguson have reached out to every farmer? Where else could he have garnered such solid grass-roots support? Where else was such a highly developed social conscience and community cooperation the basis of every day life? As Premier T.C. Douglas said at the fiftieth anniversary of the founding of the League, Saskatchewan people had developed "a special capacity to meet and solve problems that by far excels more fortunate places."

Ferguson's Credentials

Ferguson's interest in research had stemmed from his student experience in Dr. S.J.S. Pierce's laboratory in Winnipeg, where typhoid vaccine was produced for the Canadian troops in World War I. His interest in tuberculosis had been stimulated by his work with Dr. Stewart at Ninette. His first year in medical practice in Winnipeg under Dr. A.B. Alexander had been the best possible preparation for his later career, with first-hand responsibility at the King George, the infectious disease hospital, and the King Edward, the city's tuberculosis hospital. His three postulates of tuberculosis control – early discovery, reduction of the level of infection in the community, and interruption of the transmission of the tubercle bacillus – became the basis for the Saskatchewan program which comprised the following: mass surveys of the healthy population, as well as travelling consultants and strategically situated outpatient clinics for examination of contacts (early detection) and of ex-patients (follow up); BCG vaccination and pasteurization of milk (prevention); adequate sanatorium beds (segregation).

Ferguson was a rare person, superb in every aspect of his work. He was not merely what modern medical colleges call a "triple threat man" with skills in teaching, clinical work, and research. He was, in fact, a "quadruple threat man" with administrative skills as well.

Moreover, he was a physician with infinite compassion. He knew exactly how to comfort the suffering, homesick and lonesome. For about one year, as the only doctor at the sanatorium, he was on call twenty-four hours a day, yet it was not unusual for him to stay up all night holding the hand of a dying patient. In his quiet way, by example and conviction, he taught all who came in contact with him and his work: doctors, nurses, medical students, patients, their families, and the general public.

The Sanatorium Opens and Expands, 1917–1923

The sanatorium opened its doors for the admission of patients on 10 October 1917. The initial plant consisted of the administration building, two pavilions, a superintendent's residence, the power house and barn.

The words "sanitarium" and "sanatorium" do not have precisely the same origin. Sanitarium, the older word, applied to health resorts, usually with beneficial mineral springs, and it was the name given to the first tuberculosis institution in Canada at Gravenhurst. However, in 1904, to emphasize the need for scientific healing, a new word was chosen, derived from the Latin verb "sanare" to heal, rather than from the previously used noun, "sanitas," meaning health. The first institution in Canada to use the new name was the Mountain Sanatorium at Hamilton, Ontario.

Staff on opening day consisted of Dr. Ferguson, medical superintendent (with a salary of $400 per month); Miss E. May Fraser, lady superintendent ($100 monthly); Mr. E.W. Miller, accountant ($1,000 per annum); nurses Miss Jenner and Miss Wynn ($65 monthly); Frank Shirtcliffe, engineer ($100 monthly); Frank Parkins and Foster Jackson, firemen. There was also a teamster. Maids received $25 monthly and orderlies $35 to $40. Soon a laundryman, Nelson P. Smith, was hired at $75 monthly and a cook at $60. There was no ceremony to mark the opening of the sanatorium – all staff members were much too busy.

Admissions to the sanatorium came slowly. Only three patients were admitted on opening day: Miss Lilly Leslie, stenographer, of Lebret; Mr. W.H. Madden, commercial traveller, Saskatoon; and Corporal Lennie, North West Mounted Police. Upon recovery, Madden worked as steward in the sanatorium. There were twenty patients at the first Hallowe'en party. Miss Jenner and Miss Wynn, the two staff nurses, wrote an appropriate verse about each patient, and the small booklet was given to Dr. Ferguson as a keepsake.

On 1 December 1917 the first six patients from the armed forces arrived, the vanguard of an almost continuous stream of soldiers who would arrive every week or so for two years. The soldiers encountered someone they had to respect. On first meeting him, they saw Ferguson as an impressive figure with a husky voice, but when they became familiar with his innate modesty and genuine kindness, they viewed him, Dr. George J. Wherrett said, as "a father-confessor and source of inspiration." By Christmas the number of patients had increased to forty. Before the end of February all seventy beds were occupied.

The Invalided Tuberculous Soldiers' Welfare League was made up of soldier patients. Affiliated with the Great War Veterans of Canada, it was eventually known as the Tuberculous Veterans' Section of the Royal Canadian Legion. Its main purpose was to assist all tuberculous veterans and their families. These enthusiastic men participated actively in many events and projects. They formed the Recreation Club to provide entertainment for patients and staff, founded the patients' library and published the *Valley Echo*, printing the first 500 copies in December 1919. The stated purpose was "the arousing of interest in the welfare and rehabilitation of those soldiers who were returning from military to civil life by way of the sanatorium; the desire to help the civilian patients who were seeking a new lease on life in the Institution; and the carrying on of an educational campaign for the prevention of tuberculosis."

Financially, the *Valley Echo* seemed to operate on faith. It was organized without capital, all services were voluntary, and expenses were paid at the end of each month from the proceeds of subscriptions and advertising. Once or twice it was reported that the paper was broke; once, that no more issues would be published. Nevertheless, subsequent numbers continued to appear for fifty years.

During Pierre Galway-Foley's tenure as editor, the paper rapidly approached the status of a first-class tabloid, as described by Ferguson in 1939:

> In it he aired his views regarding the patients, the staff and the administration of the League, in a manner that *Hush* [an irreverent satirical magazine of the time] might have envied. His wit, combined with his facility for presenting events and personalities, resulted in a sporadic increase in circulation. On the day when The *Valley Echo* was due back from press a large crowd would gather to await its arrival and in a very short time the entire issue would be sold out . . . Those whose names had been omitted breathed a sigh of relief; those whose peccadillos had been brought into the limelight vowed vengeance, yet no one found grounds for libel.

By May 1920 it cost $110 to publish one issue and League support became necessary. The League agreed to purchase 200 copies monthly at ten cents per copy, and to distribute these to municipalities which had patients in the sanatorium. As the soldier population diminished, the Recreation Club took over publication and the League increased its support to $50 per month, Ferguson recognizing the value of the publication for education and morale-building. Remembering Pauline Johnson and her celebrated poem "The Legend of the Qu'Appelle Valley," Ferguson said, "There is something about the environs of the Qu'Appelle Valley which stimulates the sojourner to expression."

In the first year everyone, except the Ferguson family, lived in the Administration Building – where initially there was no heat. The main boilers had not arrived. Each resident purchased a small coal oil stove in an attempt to keep warm. On Saturdays, once the boilers had been installed they had to be cleaned; even the Infirmary was without heat and the nurses had to provide gallons of warming soup for the patients and themselves. Most of the nurses came from Winnipeg. When Dr. Ferguson and Miss Fraser extended an invitation to the staff, "No one thought of saying 'No.'"

Everyone worked a ten-hour day, from 7:00 a.m. to 7:00 p.m., with two hours off. Dr. Ferguson was on twenty-four-hour call. There was only one telephone at first, so a nurse or orderly would walk to the house on the hill to fetch him whenever he was needed. Staff and patients ate in the large dining room, but at separate tables. Before a meal everyone gathered in the assembly room, and for nearly a year the nurses did not allow anyone to go into the main dining room until Dr. Ferguson had arrived to lead the way.

Each Monday morning after breakfast, patients not confined to bed met in the assembly room where health instruction was given before each was weighed. Ferguson would talk about "cough," "food for recovery," "the dangers of over-exercise," "making the most of the cure hour," and "how to protect others from infection." They were taught moderation in everything except rest. To walk "slow and lazy" was the ideal; some patients mastered this for life.

During 1918 four pavilions were added for adults, which trebled the capacity to accommodate 260 patients.

Ferguson was the acting medical superintendent, filling in for Lieutenant-Colonel William Malloch Hart of the Canadian Army Medical Corps. He knew he would have to step down to the position of assistant director when Hart returned as medical director. On 8 March 1918 the League wrote to Dr. Hart "pointing out the necessity of making a permanent appointment by July 1918" and asking whether "he was in a position to return to Canada to resume duties by that date." A decision was urgent, because the League hoped to appoint a second medical doctor to assist Dr. Ferguson. Meanwhile a patient, Frank Burton Walsh, demobilized to the sanatorium with a chest lesion thought to be active tuberculosis (which, in fact, was only a scar from a war injury), had been engaged on 10 October 1918 as Ferguson's temporary assistant at $100 monthly. Walsh, a bright and enthusiastic medical student from Queen's University, soon left to complete his medical training at Winnipeg. (Later, at Johns Hopkins University, Walsh became the world's foremost neuro-ophthalmologist, author of the three-volume treatise *Clinical Neuro-ophthalmology*.)

Ferguson wrote to other sanatoria to ascertain whether any doctor interested in tuberculosis might be available as an assistant, and what salary he might expect. Nothing came of his inquiries but at least he was forearmed with physician salary schedules ($50 to $150 per month) and nurse salary schedules ($50 to $75 per month) from elsewhere in Canada.

Dr. W.M. Hart did not make up his mind quickly, nor did he return after his demobilization. He had won the Military Cross and had been mentioned in dispatches before he was taken prisoner at the second battle of Ypres. He was repatriated before the end of the war. In 1918 he became superintendent of the Special Canadian Hospital for Tuberculosis in Lenham, Kent, and was promoted to lieutenant-colonel. Finally, he returned to Canada and on 25 November 1919 submitted his resignation to Sheriff Cook, president of the League. He felt it was in the best interests of his little daughter that he should return to England. The daughter had leukemia and died in Britain. Ferguson was now appointed medical director.

Upon Hart's second return to Canada after the death of his daughter, he became a member of the Board of Sanatorium Consultants who visited all Canadian sanatoria, and a consultant to the Department of Soldiers' Civil Re-establishment (DSCR) at Ottawa. His health was greatly impaired by his war experiences and he died on 17 April 1923 in Ottawa. He was buried with full military honours in Winnipeg nine days later.

Arrival of Two Doctors and Postwar Building

In 1919, a recreation building with canteen, library, reading rooms, lounge, billiard room and auditorium was constructed. There was now an x-ray technician and a laboratory assistant. The nursing staff consisted of a matron and fourteen graduate nurses. Treatment had been given to 703 patients. The regular staff complement was augmented by members of the "vocational department" of the federal DSCR.

Dr. Robert Wellesley Kirkby arrived on 1 February, at a salary of $1,800 per year with board. After service in the Canadian Army, he had received his M.D. from Queen's University. During his internship in Vancouver he had received a letter from his former classmate, Frank B. Walsh, asking whether he could come to help Dr. Ferguson, who was overworked because of the severe influenza epidemic. Although Kirkby came on a three-month appointment, certain influences caused him to stay. "Even in my days in high school in North Battleford," he explained, "five of the boys I went to school with died of TB before they reached manhood. So I had a grudge against TB. When I saw what kind of a man Dr. Ferguson was, I decided I was going to stick with him." And the nurses were attractive. On 1 August 1919 he accepted a one-year appointment at $2,400, and a year later, when his salary was raised to $3,000 with residence supplied, he thought it was time to marry one of the nurses, Marie Berg.

Dr. Harvey Crawford Boughton accepted a position at the sanatorium for nine months, beginning 1 August 1919, at $225 monthly. Born in Arden, Manitoba, on 16 April 1889, he obtained his M.D. from the University of Manitoba in 1914. While in Yorkton, where he looked after the practice of Dr. Frank J. Irving, who was serving overseas, Dr. Boughton had on several occasions come to relieve Dr. Ferguson during the severe influenza epidemic of 1918. The two men worked well together. After one year, he received a raise to $3,000, with residence supplied, and was given the title of assistant medical superintendent.

Dr. Ferguson summarized his perception of the institution in his report at the end of 1919:

> The sanatorium idea in this province has scarcely taken form. The prestige and traditions of an institution are its chief assets. There is the indefinable something that impresses one on entering or visiting an institution and which embraces its traditions, its atmosphere, its spirit, its life. When we think of the future of this institution we do not think of its buildings and equipment, but rather of an idea, a force, a group of associations, and locality with hopeful traditions, glowing with prestige and confidence in the cure of a disease.
>
> We would like to think of it first as a medical centre, where is available every facility for the diagnosis and treatment of tuberculosis, where a sick man may get every chance to regain his broken health and return to the fullest possible sphere of usefulness as a citizen.
>
> We want it secondly to be an educational centre where the facts about a disease are being accumulated for public use; a centre where sufferers may come to get an education in regard to a disease, may learn its cure and prevention.
>
> Last of all, we want it to have the atmosphere of a home. A home where those who have fallen ill with the disease may come to rest and receive the encouragement and direction necessary to win a hard fight, and a home to which they may afterwards return to be built up, should they become run down,

or be deprived of their resistance through an acute illness or other misfortune.

On Christmas day the doctors and nurses made rounds, taking time to chat and admire gifts, in no apparent hurry to join their own families. New Year's Day was the time of the annual staff banquet and dance. Everyone gathered in the assembly room. Dr. Ferguson and his wife started up the room on one side and down the other, shaking hands and wishing each up-patient a Happy New Year. The banquet was an exceptional meal, beginning with grapefruit cocktail and ending with ice cream, coffee and salted nuts, with turkey and trimmings in between. Dr. Ferguson always gave the main speech. Dr. Boughton's orchestra played and everyone sang.

A sixteen-page booklet published early in 1920 described the sanatorium. The $80,000 fireproof administration building, built of brick and reinforced concrete, contained the offices, examination rooms, laboratory, x-ray department, kitchens, store rooms, nurses' quarters and "rooms for help." The $85,000 fireproof infirmary, built of tile and reinforced concrete, with stucco finish, accommodated eighty patients. Half of the rooms were single bedrooms. In addition, there were isolation wards, an operating theatre, chart room and examination room. Rooms on the south side connected to sleeping balconies and those on the north to summer porches, for patients inconvenienced by the summer heat. There were two $25,000 pavilions of twenty-four beds and four $32,000 pavilions of thirty-two beds. All buildings were steam-heated from a central power house. There were barns for milking cows, a piggery, a poultry ranch and a five-acre garden.

The booklet invited the public to visit and learn about the "diagnostic, curative, educational, and research aims" of the sanatorium, saying that "in tuberculosis lies dormant, yet persistent and menacing, the greatest threat to the existence of the human race."

Prospective patients were offered advice:

> Those who feel unable personally to bear the expense of treatment should obtain from the local reeve, mayor or overseer, a certificate assuming liability for the cost of treatment by their municipality, town or village, as provided by section 9, chapter 10, statutes of Saskatchewan, 1910–11 . . . Patients will be met at the station by the Sanatorium bus . . . Patients are expected to

> supply their own clinical thermometers and cheese cloth for handkerchiefs. These may be procured on the premises at cost . . . 'the cure' is not a bottle of medicine, nor a surgical operation, but an Idea: a way of life, to apply to every moment of the day, every activity . . . part of the cure is the development of a spirit of faithful endeavour, helpfulness, earnestness, good humour, kindliness and forbearance.

Regular visiting hours were from 4:00 p.m. to 5.00 p.m. and from 7:00 p.m. to 8:30 p.m., but visitors from a distance were accorded special privileges. Since the condition of the patient determined the number of visitors and length of visit, it was necessary to receive permission for each occasion. Tours of the San could be arranged by appointment.

The sanatorium became the main fund-raising objective for a number of provincial groups. The Imperial Order of the Daughters of the Empire (IODE) raised $45,000 to build the children's pavilion, which was opened 30 October 1919. The IODE refurbished the adjoining pavilion to expand the space to seventy children's beds, furnished the schoolroom, provided books for the school library, paid the bills of many children until treatment became free, and built the Preventorium, which opened in 1927. The IODE regent was the wife of W.M. Martin, Saskatchewan's premier. The Provincial Council of Women in 1921 launched a $50,000 drive to pay for sanatorium care for mothers with tuberculosis. The Red Cross similarly provided $16,000 to build the Red Cross Lodge, which opened on 8 October 1919 with fourteen rooms for visitors. Within a stone's throw of the sanatorium, yet almost out of sight behind a pleasant screen of trees, its large windows were said to "preach a silent but none-the-less impressive sermon on the value of fresh air."

By the end of 1921, there had been added a laundry, a $16,000 superintendent's residence, first occupied by A.B. Cook and in later years by the Ferguson family, and seven cottages for married staff. The nurses' home, completed early in 1922, had three floors, with a large and spacious balcony opening off each floor. The front door led to a fine reception room, set off by an open hearth. (This building was converted to a pavilion when a larger nurses' residence was completed in 1926, the last new building for another eighteen years.)

An outdoor bandstand was added in 1923. Open-air church services were held from the bandstand during the summer. Concerts by the

Boy Scouts' Band of Regina, the Queen City Classics, and Dr. Boughton's sanatorium orchestra were featured the first summer.

X-rays

The increasing use of radiology gradually removed most of the guesswork from the diagnosis of pulmonary tuberculosis. The first x-ray machine was purchased after the sanatorium had been in operation for seventeen months. H. Spencer Uren was sent away for a week to learn its operation and began taking exposures in March 1919. By the end of 1919, 555 exposures had been made, and 2,043 in 1920. The sanatorium at Ninette, Manitoba, also installed its first x-ray machine in 1919, after eleven years without one.

At first each chest radiograph was exposed on a large fourteen-by-seventeen-inch glass plate. Viewing and storing problems were prodigious. The glass plates were not only expensive, but cumbersome, heavy and fragile!

Strangely, there is no mention in the League minutes or in the *Valley Echo* of the epochal switch-over from glass plates to the much thinner, lighter, more flexible and more convenient x-ray films. This event probably took place late in 1919. The early films weren't without their shortcomings, however – on a cellulose nitrate base, they were highly flammable. In the Cleveland Clinic fire of 1930, many people died, thereby hastening conversion to use of a film with a cellulose acetate base, called "safety film," safe to store in buildings housing patients.

Whether the image is registered on a glass plate or a film, the earliest lesions of tuberculosis are microscopic in size and therefore invisible. Later enlargement leads to the discovery of the first barely visible "soft lesions" that allow only a tentative diagnosis. Commonly, a single film was inadequate, but a change noted between two consecutive films, three to six months apart, would be definitive.

Sanatorium Staff

Dr. Thomas Wilfred "Tommy" Hamilton, the fourth medical doctor, joined the staff on 5 December 1921, only months after his graduation from the University of Manitoba. George J. Wherrett interned at the San in December 1922 and in the summer of 1923 and joined the medical staff in January 1924. Miss Maude Montgomery was the "lady superintendent" (appointed on 15 August 1919); A.B. Cook, managing director; E.H. Southam, chief accountant; W.H. Madden, steward; R.D. Roberts, store accountant; Miss Hunter, dietitian (1 January 1921). As of early 1923 there were sixteen graduate nurses, three undergraduate nurses, eight nursing assistants, seven housekeepers, four orderlies, three technicians, four stenographers, a telephone operator, a store clerk, seventeen Chinese cooks and kitchen attendants, five engineers, four firemen, seven house cleaners, eleven house maids, one laundry manager, seven laundry employees, two seamstresses, two chauffeurs, two painters, two plumbers, two gardeners, one carpenter, one canteen steward, one teamster, one animal attendant, and two general duty men. The Red Cross Society paid the salary of the matron of the Red Cross Lodge. All told, there was one employee for every two patients, whereas in institutions fifty years later this ratio tended to be reversed. On 1 April 1920 all nurses with ten months' service received a raise to $75 a month.

There were some growing pains, with three contentious issues reaching the board of directors. The engineer was dismissed on 16 March 1921 after a discrepancy of $50 was discovered in estimates he provided for a plumbing contract. Upon hearing particulars of the lack of harmony between the steward and the secretary, the board placed the responsibility for the future conduct of the sanatorium squarely upon the shoulders of Mr. A.B. Cook, who had been appointed general manager in April 1922. "If personal or petty differences interfere . . . it will be the duty of the general manager to suspend any member or members of the staff pending the decision of the board." The third contentious issue concerned a nurse whose mother asked that she be on full pay during treatment for tuberculosis incurred on duty while the nurses' quarters had often been without heat. This nurse had received pay for 331 days and treatment for 151 days. The League responded by formulating the following policy: "In the event of illness of any of the employees of three months' service or more, they be carried on the payroll for a period not exceeding one month, and in the event of the illness being tuberculosis that they be given treatment free of charge."

With these teething troubles behind it, the institution settled down to operate for the most part as one big, happy family. The doctors and nurses lived on the grounds. Everyone faced the same enemy: tuberculosis. To fight it, they rallied behind Dr. Ferguson.

Life at Fort San, 1919–1925

The name of "Fort Qu'Appelle Sanatorium" quickly became shortened in local usage to "Fort San." Consequently Fort San became the official name for the post office, which opened on 20 December 1926.

Veterans and Their Financial Impact

Not only the needs of the returning veterans made federal money available for buildings, but the per diem allowance for treatment of veterans was sufficiently generous that the sanatorium ran into few financial difficulties so long as soldiers were present in large numbers. The Dominion Department of Soldiers' Civil Re-establishment (DSCR) at one time paid for three-quarters of the operating expenses.

In 1919, returned soldiers with tuberculosis outnumbered civilian patients by three to one. For every 100 soldiers who died in action, another 6 died of tuberculosis. Of every 100 servicemen discharged on a pension, 25 received theirs for tuberculosis. There were 769 admissions of returned men to the Fort Qu'Appelle Sanatorium between 1917 and 1925. Their median age on admission was thirty-two, but the median age of the 23 percent who died was only twenty-five years and six months.

In spite of the expectation that on enlistment soldiers should have been healthier than average, tuberculosis was twice as common among veterans as it was among civilians of the same age. The high rate of infection was attributed to hardships of service, exposure to intercurrent infections and close contact with tubercular victims at the barracks. One-quarter of the men admitted to the San with tuberculosis had been exposed to German poisonous chlorine gas at Ypres on 22 April 1915, or in later attacks, to mustard gas (dichlorethyl sulfide). Sixty percent of those exposed were returned to Canada and half were still disabled at the end of the war.

The returned soldiers presented difficulties in discipline rarely seen with civilians. They had been looking forward to freedom from army discipline, but at the sanatorium they came up against rules which were even more restrictive. Some of them rebelled. Ferguson had infinite sympathy and patience, but he did insist that the rules be enforced for the patients' own good.

Like many soldiers, Ferguson was a cigarette smoker, but he soon switched to a pipe. Although the *Valley Echo*, as early as 1924, carried warnings about the danger of smoking for patients with tuberculosis, cigarettes were sold in the canteen and advertised in the *Valley Echo*. (By contrast, Ninette Sanatorium had rules restricting smoking to after meals and before bedtime, and did not sell tobacco in the canteen.)

As the percentage of soldiers decreased, the substantial amount of "sure money" was replaced by "uncertain money" from a motley group of sources. In 1924, for example, Ferguson had to arrange payment from twelve sources for the 295 patients under treatment at the end of the year.

Table 1

League Sources of Money in 1924

	Number of Patients
Municipal pool	70
DSCR for veterans	48
Rural municipalities	44
Cities and towns	20
Private payment by patient	29
Department of Indian Affairs	26
Every Woman's Fund	12
Free treatment fund for children	10
Department of Public Health	10
Department of Municipal Affairs	5
Sanatorium staff	1
No definite arrangement	20
Total	**295**

Thus, only 29 of 295 individuals with a chronic illness requiring an average of one year's treatment could pay the full fee of $2.50 per day. The government's grant of fifty cents per patient-day was identical to that paid for patients in general hospitals.

Entertainment

Entertainment, whether provided from within or from outside, was a great booster of patient morale. An orchestra began modestly in 1919 when Dr. Boughton and others gave several selections at a concert. Its formal debut came during the intermission of a play staged by the Dramatic Club in February 1920. Dr. Boughton remained the conductor of the eighteen to twenty-two players until he left for Saskatoon. Ambulant patients were allowed to play string instruments but wind instruments were proscribed.

Many volunteer groups came to provide entertainment. On 28 December 1922, for example, a party of collegiate students from Yorkton, under their teacher, P. Dallin, with Professor T.A. George as their musical director, put on an entertaining musical comedy, "Betty's Dilemma." One of the students, Leon Edel, who later became famous as the biographer of Henry James, played violin solos and was reported to be "one of Saskatchewan's premier violinists." Leon Edel describes the experience: "I remember it as if it were yesterday: the cold clear weather, the long corridors, the applause, and the underpinning of sadness I experienced at the thought of all those patients confined by their tuberculosis. It must have chimed in with my high adolescence. I was fifteen, and as addicted to music then as I am to letters [now]."

Only limited outdoor activities were possible. An autumn corn roast often celebrated the joint twelfth of September birthdays of Ferguson and Kirkby. Lawn croquet was popular. The sanatorium bus and the famous motorboat, "Minnie-ha-ha," were piloted by a veteran with a distinguished war record, Wallace S. Stiff, known as "Stiffy." Stiff later became the undertaker. Indoors, there were whist and bridge parties and cribbage tournaments. Silent movies and, later, sound movies were shown weekly. Reading, of course, was the salvation of a number of patients. The nucleus of the library at Fort San was a set of 350 books brought by the returned soldiers from the temporary hospital quarters in Regina. By June 1920 there were about 1,500 books, and by April 1921, 2,000 books. The library was run by the patients.

The in-house journal, *Valley Echo*, was popular, even with readers who were not bookworms. This unpretentious little monthly paper encouraged contributions from any patient.

But the great success at Fort San was the introduction of the radio. Milton Russell in pavilion "31" and Jimmy Cooke in "24" each had a radio set. After the earphones came loudspeakers. Because the man down the corridor could not stretch his exercise to come to the loudspeaker, Russell rigged up an extension for earphones; the next step was to try two sets of earphones, and when it worked, the idea spread like wildfire and the whole floor of the pavilion was hooked up.

One night in January 1923, Jimmy led a wire from his set into Hazel Hart's room on the floor below. She later claimed this was the first extension from one floor to another for any sanatorium in the world. By spring every patient in the pavilion was connected to his or her own set. The next step was to connect up a neighbouring pavilion.

Russell's antenna was elevated thirty-five feet and was grounded to a radiator. He made his connection to the Infirmary, 300 feet away, using an overhead twisted wire. Altogether over 3,000 feet of no. 18 wire were run along the balcony on porcelain knobs and brought down to connections at each bed. Despite the enormous resistance of the eighty headsets, all in series, only seventy-two volts on the plate were necessary to give plenty of volume to signals all along the line.

As Hazel Hart reported in the *Valley Echo*:

> The [Regina] Leader-Post Broadcasting Station, CKCK, put on a campaign, with an appeal from His Honour the Lieutenant Governor, to provide a head set for each patient, and were completely successful, to the great delight of every patient . . . Sanatoria all across Canada . . . wrote to Doctor Ferguson for plans of our set-up . . . Our Sanatorium physicians feel that radio is one of their strongest allies. Otherwise restless patients will lie quietly for hours listening to their favorite programs . . . their diseased lungs are given that much better opportunity to heal.

Commitment to Postgraduate Education

Ferguson was one of the first sanatorium administrators in Canada to give a high priority to continuing education. Even when the San was hopelessly in debt during years of drought and depression, even when short-handed during wartime, Ferguson sent his staff away to learn. Because of the excellent and renowned teachers and the wealth of clinical experience available, and in spite of the time and expense to get there, London, England, was one of the most popular destinations. Training could be rewarded by success at the MRCP examination. Members of the medical staff often took an entire year of postgraduate training at the sanatorium's expense; over the years, this proved to be a good investment. Radiographers, nurses and dietitians were regularly sent away for short courses and practical experience in another institution. There was no requirement of years of service to become eligible. If the sanatorium needed someone trained in a new technique, and if there was a young staff member eager to learn, an educational opportunity was available after only one or two years at the sanatorium.

Boughton was the first to take educational leave; he spent two weeks in Winnipeg in 1920. Ferguson then went to Boston for two months late in 1920; he spent one month studying heart disease with Dr. Paul White, a world-renowned cardiologist, and three weeks taking a

$100 course in internal medicine at Harvard University. Ferguson found that the physician who is limited to treating one disease "is apt to develop a blind side, and to lose his true perspective in the interpretation of symptoms which are the common stock of widely different diseases." To recognize early tuberculosis, one had to keep in touch with the whole field of internal medicine. At Boston, which was one of the first centres to provide clinics for graduates in medicine and which had a splendid medical library, a doctor's medical experience and perspectives could be broadened. Each year at least one sanatorium physician went away for special studies.

School at the Sanatorium

Long-term treatment of children raised the question of their schooling. Must children fall behind in their schooling or could instruction be provided in the sanatorium? Ferguson, committed to education, made every effort to ensure that children received as much instruction as was compatible with their treatment.

Formal schooling began in the children's pavilion on 13 January 1921, with Miss Ethel M. Bolton, B.A., as the first teacher. In January 1922, Gertrude Ketchen took over. After her marriage to Robert Connell, she described her "four very happy and rewarding years" in this way:

> Classes began at 8.30 a.m. till 10.30 a.m., followed by the rest period; the afternoon session began at 2.30 p.m. and lasted until 4.00 p.m. . . . arranged so as not to conflict with the medical treatment of the children. All the eligible pupils began with one-half hour instruction and gradually worked up to the maximum of two hours per day . . . The children looked forward to attending classes.
>
> During my second teaching year . . . the idea of bedside teaching was formed. At least three pupils completed their grade eight departmental examinations . . . two of them went on through high school and subsequently became teachers.

To be a teacher required unusual dedication and an ability to improvise and inspire. The days were long. A few years later the teacher at the Saskatoon San, Jean Cocks, had the habit of going back to the wards at 8.15 p.m. to hear the children say their prayers.

— Chapter Four —

Baseline Studies, 1921–1924

FERGUSON HAD A practical, common-sense approach as he planned his assault on tuberculosis. He needed to assess the magnitude of the problem. No other jurisdiction in North America had cross-sectional school and Normal School surveys to equal his, and no other sanatorium system kept better statistics to follow the course of later progress. Financing for such studies would have been an almost insuperable problem if it had not been for the establishment of the Saskatchewan Anti-tuberculosis Commission, which, in 1921, made possible the eight-community cross-sectional school survey and the questionnaire survey of all practising medical doctors. After the commission had reported in October 1922, Ferguson felt there was still a need for a survey of the children of one entire community, and he persuaded the Weyburn Rotary Club to provide the money and much of the manpower for the Weyburn survey of 1924.

The Saskatchewan Anti-tuberculosis Commission

The Saskatchewan Anti-tuberculosis Commission, often incorrectly called "the Royal Commission," was established by order-in-council, 22 July 1921, "to enquire into the question of tuberculosis in the province." A.B. Cook of Regina, the chairman of the Saskatchewan Anti-tuberculosis League, was the chairman; Dr. Ferguson organized the investigations and wrote the final report; R.H. Brighton of Regina, a former patient and co-editor of the *Valley Echo*, was the secretary, but did not sign the final report; and J.F. Cairns, a prominent businessman from Saskatoon, was the fourth member.

Five thousand information pamphlets were printed and distributed to ex-patients of the sanatorium; to reeves, councillors and secretary-treasurers of municipalities, city councils, hospital boards, and school boards; to medical health officers; and to all physicians.

The Eight-Community Cross-sectional School Survey, 1921

In the 1921 cross-sectional survey, arrangements were made with the school boards to examine about 200 selected children between the ages of six and fourteen in each of eight representative communities: Regina, Saskatoon, Moose Jaw, North Battleford, Cupar, Stoughton and Heward. The children were tuberculin-tested and there was simultaneous tuberculin-testing of cattle in the same areas.

The surveys were done with a degree of informed consent that was imperfect by modern standards, yet somewhat advanced for the time. Each parent received the following notice from the secretary of the school board:

> The object of these tests is to ascertain as nearly as possible the percentage of school children affected with any physical or clinical defects that are liable to encourage the development of tuberculosis. All school examinations will be carried out under the direction of R.G. Ferguson, Superintendent of the Saskatchewan Sanatorium. The school your child is attending has been selected for examination.
>
> If you have any objection to having your child included in the group inspected, please sign the attached form and return to the teacher. If the form is not signed and returned, it will be understood that you have given your consent to the examination.

The examinations were carried out between Monday and Friday by four nurses, two chest specialists, a dentist and two ear, nose and throat specialists. Each child was weighed and given a tuberculin test. The afternoon temperature and pulse were recorded and teeth and tonsils examined. A home survey of economic living conditions and health of families was carried out at the same time. The results were interesting:

- Ten of 1,184 (nearly 1 percent) children examined had active tuberculosis; another fifteen were found from a follow-up radiograph to have tuberculosis. Radiographs were obtained for only eighty children.
- A positive tuberculin test in 56.6 percent of children indicated that they had already been infected (44 percent were positive by age six and 61 percent by age fourteen); there was little difference between boys and girls.
- A positive tuberculin test was present in 75.6 percent of Normal School students; 0.9 percent had active tuberculosis.
- A positive tuberculin test was present in 93.1 percent of the 162 Indian children examined in residential schools.
- Of 185 dairy cows given tuberculin, 34 (18.5 percent) tested positive.

  Children in areas with the highest percentage of tuberculous cows had the highest percentage of positive tuberculin tests, about triple the positive rate in the cows.
- As to general health, 10.3 percent of the white children were judged to be undernourished, 47.1 percent had one or more decaying teeth, 25.3 percent had diseased tonsils and 18.8 percent had excessive adenoid tissue. The tuberculin-positive rate was 11 percent higher in the 9.4 percent of children who came from "poor homes."

This was important information, useful for future comparisons.

Public Hearings

Public hearings, although not then a common procedure, were held in all seven cities and in Yorkton, which was to become Saskatchewan's eighth city a few years later. Many who appeared before the commission represented local government or hospital boards. The four specific questions and the consensus of the replies were as follows:

> Q. Should tuberculosis patients be treated in general hospitals, or should they be cared for in institutions specially designed and equipped for the purpose?

A. The unanimous view was that special hospitals (sanatoria) were required to provide more specialized treatment with better discipline, and to reduce the danger of cross-infection to other patients in the general hospital.

Q. How should the cost for necessary buildings, equipment and treatment be apportioned as between municipalities, the provincial government, and the patient?
A. The consensus was that the cost of buildings and equipment should be borne by the province at large, since all communities would benefit.

Q. What responsibility should the municipality be required to assume with respect to its own tuberculous residents?
A. Most respondents felt that the patient should pay, when able to do so, but that the cost should be borne by the municipality and the provincial government when the patient could not pay. The municipal representatives, however, told of cases where the municipality, after giving aid, had seized land and chattels for reimbursement, leaving the family with insufficient support. Further, municipalities were responsible for the support of indigent patients only after thirty days residence; those unable to work gravitated to the cities, which then assumed a disproportionate burden.

Q. What responsibility should the provincial government be required to assume in order to assist in providing treatment for tuberculous patients?
A. Most responded that it was fairer, and best for the maintenance of the public's health, if the provincial government assumed a greater role in paying health care costs of indigents.

The Commission Report

The ninety-four-page report of the survey, published in October 1922, consisted of three main parts: general information, results of the surveys of prevalence, and a series of recommendations for the future.

General Information

After reiterating many points of general information, the report pointed out:

- The greatest danger to the public is the careless cougher and spitter.
- Many are in the advanced stage before they realize they have the disease.
- The undernourished child is especially susceptible.

The commission interviewed many patients, individually and in groups. The reasons given for the disease having reached an advanced state before treatment was sought included:

- Difficulty in accurate diagnosis by family physicians.
- Reluctance to admit the presence of tuberculosis.
- Inadequate personal finances and reluctance to apply for municipal charity.
- Unwillingness of patients, especially mothers, to travel far from their homes and families for the length of time required to effect a complete cure.

Saskatchewan, Indians excepted, conquered the dreaded tuberculosis much earlier than Great Britain. In Britain, as late as 1934, fear, a sense of fatalism, the social stigma attached to the disease, the prospect of supervision, the threatened invasion of the home by the authorities, and the fear of unemployment and financial hardship if the disease was discovered, were still cited as reasons for delay in seeking medical advice. Poverty, overcrowding and malnutrition favoured tuberculosis, which in turn led to more poverty. Britain was also slow to control bovine tuberculosis and to pasteurize milk. In Saskatchewan, the vicious circle of poverty and tuberculosis was eliminated among Caucasians but has persisted among Indians.

There were thirty-seven hospitals with 1,614 beds in Saskatchewan. Only thirty-two patients with tuberculosis were being treated in these hospitals, in spite of a provincial requirement that 10 percent of bed capacity be set aside for tuberculosis patients.

Other Surveys

Other studies carried out by the commission revealed:

- The Military Draft Board in 1918 had rejected 1.9 percent of recruits because of active tuberculosis.

- Of all mothers receiving aid under the Mothers' Pension Act, 57 of 436 respondents were widowed by reason of tuberculosis and 12 of these mothers themselves had active disease. In these 57 households there had already been 143 deaths from tuberculosis, and there were now 63 active cases of tuberculosis, including 27 children.
- Physicians had 1,625 patients with tuberculosis under their care, clearly indicating a serious shortage of beds in the sanatorium.
- The average sanatorium stay was only 5.4 months (4.3 months for civilians and 7.15 months for service veterans for whom money was guaranteed by the federal government).
- Sixty-eight percent of patients left the sanatorium before their disease was arrested and 75 percent were unable to pay for their treatment.
- No follow-up clinics were available.

Recommendations of the Commission

Of the commission's recommendations, the first four (boldface type), were considered mandatory and twelve (asterisks) were soon implemented.

* **Hospital and sanatorium accommodation must be increased to care for those who are spreaders of the disease.** [The commission recommended the construction of two new sanatoria of at least one hundred beds each, to allow each patient twelve months of treatment.]

* **There must be provision for the care of children from homes where open tuberculosis is found.** A preventorium should be established to prevent the newborn infant from contracting tuberculosis from its mother. Children, especially those under three, should be separated from actively tuberculous parents.

* **The system of financing the cost of treatment must enable all those who need treatment to obtain it with the least delay.** The proportion of the cost to be borne by the province and by the municipality for the treatment of those who could not pay was not yet defined.

* **Diagnostic facilities must be improved and extended to all parts of the province, along with a nursing service and follow-up of all ex-tuberculous patients.** Free diagnostic and follow-up clin-

ics, staffed by nurses and tuberculosis specialists, should begin at the two centres with adequate laboratories, Saskatoon and the Fort Qu'Appelle Sanatorium.

* A travelling specialist should be provided to assist physicians in outlying districts.
* Federal authorities should make a complete survey of the Indian population, make special provisions to prevent the spread of tuberculosis among them, and test cattle on Indian reserves for bovine tuberculosis.
* All cows supplying milk to children should be tested for tuberculosis; accredited tuberculosis-free herd areas should be established.
* Each student nurse should receive training in the prevention and management of tuberculosis.
* Postgraduate training in tuberculosis should be provided for physicians who desire it.
* Health should be taught in schools, with special reference to tuberculosis. Normal School students should be given special instruction concerning the prevention, early symptoms and management of tuberculosis. Each public health nurse should take a postgraduate course at the sanatorium.
* Laboratories should be provided for bacteriologic examinations.
* Meat inspection should be provided at all abattoirs and slaughter houses to prevent the distribution of tuberculous meat.

- General hospitals of fifty beds or more should temporarily assign 10 percent of their beds for tuberculous patients, and receive the same remuneration per patient-day as the sanatorium.
- Every food handler should possess a certificate of good health.
- Tuberculosis should be made a quarantinable disease as soon as the necessary accommodation for open cases has been provided, the quarantine to be applied only if the patient fails to cooperate. This should be combined with compulsory reporting of each person with tuberculosis.
- There should be one public health nurse for each 1,000 school children.
- Homes should be completely disinfected following removal of a patient with open tuberculosis.
- All school children should be examined to identify those with

active tuberculosis, to eliminate sources of infection and to identify any predisposing causes.

- Underweight children should be in sunny ungraded classrooms with a south exposure and open windows in all but extreme weather, and have an hour of complete rest during both forenoon and afternoon, together with a glass of milk each time.
- Complete ventilation of theatres and public halls should be required.
- Convalescent vocational training should be provided at Fort Qu'Appelle.

The commission also made a strong statement on government financing, which they agreed was necessary for most capital expenditures and for a substantial proportion of the cost of treatment. They felt, however, that total government control would be disastrous. If all work were undertaken by government and paid for by a general tax, it would make things easier to manage, but "many necessary elements" would entirely disappear, since the public would feel there was nothing left for them to do, and the educational advantages of fund-raising campaigns would be lost. Members of the League were "rendering voluntary services to the sufferers with tuberculosis that could not be purchased with money."

The Weyburn Survey, 1924

There had been 125 deaths from tuberculosis among Saskatchewan children under five years of age in the previous five years, one-quarter of these attributed to milk. The statistics provided Ferguson's motivation for the Weyburn survey, supported financially by the Weyburn Rotary Club and believed to be the first comprehensive health survey of all school children in any North American community. Ann Morton of the Weyburn Board of Education was in charge of planning and acted as secretary of the Health Survey Committee. The survey began on 22 September 1924.

The doctors taking part in the Weyburn school survey were R.G. Ferguson, R.W. Kirkby, T.W. Hamilton, H.S. Good and Sigga Christianson. Robert Connell took the radiographs, assisted by Miss Hall. The Saskatchewan Department of Public Health supplied two nurses, Mrs. Bennett and Miss Peers. The school hygiene branch of the Department of Education provided Miss MacDonald and Miss Chittick.

Local volunteers included Nurse Bell, Nurse Matheson, Miss Irmie, Miss Kemp and a number of female collegiate students. The physicians and dentists of Weyburn and the doctors at the mental hospital donated their services.

The x-ray machine was provided free by Mr. W.M. Martin of Victor X-ray Corporation, Winnipeg. Every child received two postero-anterior stereoscopic exposures and a lateral exposure, for a total of three films, a thoroughness which was most unusual for that era.

The purpose was to ascertain the prevalence of tuberculosis in children. Only 0.2 percent had tuberculosis of the lymph nodes, while 0.8 percent had active pulmonary infection requiring treatment. Another 3.8 percent had evidence of pulmonary tuberculosis, perhaps inactive, but requiring continued, regular observation. A positive tuberculin test, indicating previous exposure to tuberculosis, was encountered in 40 percent of children.

Few children were perfectly healthy. The doctors recorded the prevalence of defective vision (23 percent), impaired hearing (2 percent), enlarged tonsils (31 percent), nasal obstruction or infection (15 percent), dental disease (poor teeth in 30 percent with one or more decayed teeth in 63 percent and gum abscess in 17 percent), goitre (4 percent), orthopaedic defects (1 percent), hernia or phimosis requiring herniorrhaphy or circumcision, respectively (6 percent) rheumatic heart disease (3 percent), kidney disease (8 percent) and undernourishment (7 percent).

Achievements of the Commission

Unlike many government surveys whose recommendations are not implemented, the first twelve recommendations of the Saskatchewan Anti-tuberculosis Commission's were achieved quickly, even if slightly behind schedule. Dr. Frances McGill was appointed as director of the Public Health Laboratory in Regina, and free examination of sputum, forwarded in special containers supplied by the League, was offered to all doctors and hospitals before the end of the year. Sputum examination over the years proved to be the most specific and cost-effective means of arriving at the diagnosis of tuberculosis.

Few medical men have had, early in their career, occasion to document the extent of a target disease and, in doing so, to realize the opportunity to set the direction of their life's work. Ferguson, with the support of other members of the committee, was able to set and promulgate his goals (including unheard-of policies such as free treatment of tuberculosis), and then had another twenty-seven years to implement them. The opportunity to direct the research and write the commission report allowed him to produce his own blueprint for action. Once the report was completed, its chairman, A.B. Cook, was co-opted to be managing director of the League as a further safeguard to ensure that recommendations would be carried out.

Among other studies arising from the report, the Normal School student surveys continued with a chest radiograph and tuberculin test carried out each year thereafter, as a means of assessing the public exposure to tuberculosis.

Clearly the Anti-tuberculosis Commission offered the most important opportunity of Ferguson's career. He seized it and carried through.

— Chapter Five —

Three Sanatoria

Saskatoon Sanatorium, 1925

FERGUSON DESERVES CREDIT for the planning of Saskatchewan's second and third sanatoria, each on a picturesque site.

The 175-bed Saskatoon Sanatorium was built near the South Saskatchewan River on the southern edge of Saskatoon. This sanatorium was compact, not spread out like the buildings at Fort San. Patients had more privacy in two-bed wards. Of steel frame construction with brick to the second-storey floor-line, it cost $512,000. Two years later, a $62,000 nurses' home was added.

Harvey Boughton was promoted from assistant superintendent at Fort San to become Saskatoon's medical superintendent, a position he held until his retirement twenty-four years later. The Saskatoon Sanatorium opened on 15 April 1925 and the next day fifty-seven patients were admitted; soon the first 135 beds were full. Miss E.E. Love, formerly assistant matron at Fort San, was the matron. R.D. Roberts took over the secretarial work. Percy Hunt was the x-ray technician. Twenty patients with tuberculosis were transferred from City and St. Paul's hospitals and another thirty-two whose homes were in the northern part of the province were moved from Fort San.

Boughton attributed his interest in tuberculosis to the excellent training he had received from Dr. David A. Stewart at Ninette during two periods of internship. One year after the opening of the new sanatorium, the University of Saskatchewan began to offer instruction in the first two years of medicine only. Boughton immediately became a part-time teacher, giving lectures at the university and demonstrating clinical signs in physical diagnosis at the sanatorium. After discovering that 4 percent of previous medical students had developed tuberculosis, Boughton vaccinated each student with BCG and taught them that a tuberculin test should be part of a physical examination.

Boughton experimented with tuberculosis surveys among schoolchildren, at the request of interested communities, conducting tuberculin and x-ray surveys with his familiar car and trailer unit. In one three-week survey, with a nurse and two x-ray technicians, he examined 12,000 individuals. Boughton's surveys led to development of the photofluorographic survey, "a method of surveying more people in a shorter time at less cost." Thus he played an important role in developing methods for early detection.

Boughton was very musical. While at college he had studied organ under Stanley Osborne. He was organist and choir master in churches wherever his medical duties took him, in Yorkton, at Fort Qu'Appelle, at the Third Avenue, Knox and St. Thomas-Wesley United churches in Saskatoon, and at Christ Church (Anglican) in Saskatoon. He was a member of the Canadian College of Organists.

He retired in April 1959 after thirty-four years of service with the League. Hazel Hart, director of Christmas Seal sales for Canada, came from the Canadian Tuberculosis Association in Ottawa for his retirement ceremonies. Boughton was first listed as editor of the *Valley Echo* in January 1960, and this became one of his main activities in retirement.

Boughton had been president of the Saskatoon and District Medical Society and of the medical staff at St. Paul's Hospital, Saskatoon. He was awarded the King George V Silver Jubilee Medal in 1935 and the George VI Coronation Medal in 1937. He was a Fellow of the Royal College of Physicians of Canada and a Senior Member of the Canadian Medical Association. For a number of years he was a member of the board of directors of the Saskatoon Public Library.

Boughton School, newly built three blocks directly west of the Saskatoon San, was named for Dr. Boughton when it was formally opened on 2 May 1962. No other honour was more appreciated than the naming of this school in the vicinity of his life's work. The motto of the school was "Fidelia Certa Merces" (Faithful work is certain to bring reward). As the population of children in the area dwindled, the school was closed in June 1983. Boughton died on 26 May 1970.

The second sanatorium to open, Saskatoon was the last to close when the last TB patient was transferred elsewhere on 26 June 1978. However, the outpatient clinic did not move to University Hospital until 14 May 1982 and the tuberculosis laboratory continued to operate in the same buildings until it finally moved to University Hospital in September 1986. After ten years as a nursing home, the attractive buildings in their well-treed setting fell to the wrecker's ball in late 1989.

Prince Albert Sanatorium, 1930

The Prince Albert Sanatorium opened on 7 January 1930. Its new medical superintendent, Dr. Robert Kirkby, achieved full operation with amazing speed. The first fifty-nine patients, transferred from Fort San, arrived at the remote railway siding near the new San when it was nearly sixty degrees below zero Fahrenheit. Within three days, Kirkby had admitted sixty-eight patients from Saskatoon and forty-five from Moose Jaw and Regina hospitals, augmented "by the arrival of various patients from the surrounding district." All 276 beds were fully occupied within a month.

The ultra-modern, $1-million building was designed to allow access to a sun balcony for every patient. Two-thirds of the balcony roof could be removed, even on a nice winter's day. Another innovation was the siting of the kitchen on the top floor, instead of having a diet kitchen on each floor. Food trays were distributed on a continuous conveyor belt.

Kirkby, strict and outspoken but always fair, was remembered for his quick wit. He spent long hours with the critically ill, both day and night. When staff shortages occurred, he helped with menial tasks, feeding a toddler, sorting the mail, or carrying trays to patients. Once he was discovered in the vegetable room peeling potatoes!

From Prince Albert, Kirkby sent survey teams through the northern half of the province, checking for new TB outbreaks and following up on discharged patients. He opened monthly clinics at North Battleford, Melfort, Tisdale and, later, Meadow Lake and Lac la Ronge. Kirkby saw patients in their own hospitals, since people weren't likely to come seventy-five miles or more to consult him.

The last sanatorium to open, Prince Albert, was, on 30 April 1961, the first to close. Kirkby had been superintendent for thirty-one years, three months and twenty-one days, and had amassed nearly forty-two years of service with the League. He continued to work part-time, relieving the Prince Albert staff doctor, Dr. Lottie Stark, whenever she took holidays or held TB clinics in the north. In this way he served the League for almost fifty-six years, possibly a world record for years of continuous service against tuberculosis.

Fort San, 1925–1930

Fort San meanwhile was operating at a capacity of 310 beds. One exciting and nearly tragic event occurred on 20 April 1927, when a fire, due to a short circuit, broke out in the basement of the Ferguson home. The occupants were awakened by the smoke, which simultaneously alerted a nurse in the children's pavilion who called the voluntary fire brigade. The family escaped. When Ferguson went back to rescue some important papers, his foot went through the floor and he almost fell into the fiery basement. Though at first the firemen felt it was a lost cause, the fire was extinguished within two hours. The contents of the basement and two main floor rooms were totally destroyed, including family portraits, and much damage was done to the whole lower floor. Repairs took more than a month.

In 1929, Ferguson appointed Dr. Tommy Hamilton (who had married A.B. Cook's daughter) as medical superintendent of Fort San, to provide the same administrative structure for each of the three sanatoria. Ferguson thereby relieved himself of much of the administrative responsibility for Fort San and freed some time for his research and for monthly visits to each of the other two sanatoria. He retained the title of director of medical services and general superintendent, with jurisdiction over all three sanatoria.

Free Treatment, 1929

Free treatment of tuberculosis, advocated in the commission report in 1922, remained the most important plank in Ferguson's platform. He worked systematically to achieve grass-roots support for the concept, so necessary before there was any hope of implementation by the government. But it took time.

When questioned by the League directors on 21 December 1920 as to the extent of the financial barrier to treatment, Ferguson replied, "We have never refused admission to any patient, either child or adult, on account of the lack of financial support, but many persons, when they

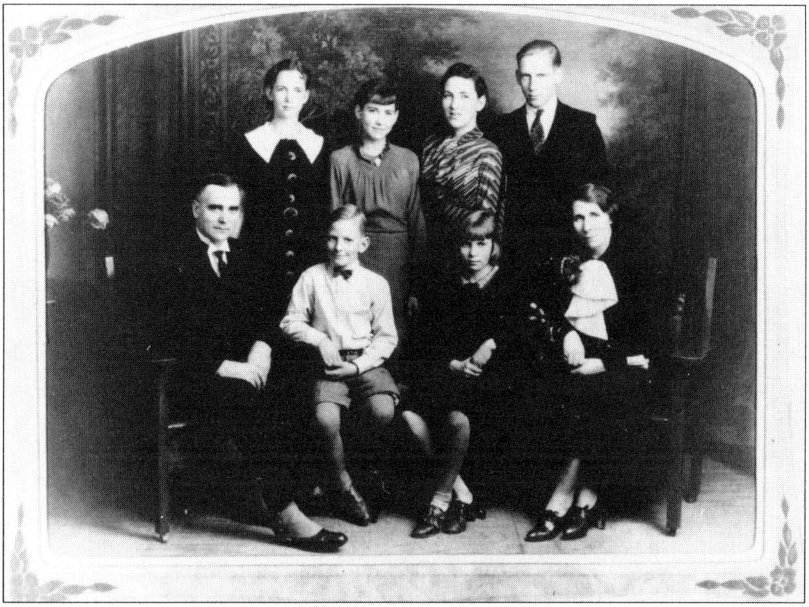

Courtesy of the Saskatchewan Lung Association

Ferguson family ca. 1935. *Back row*: Margaret, Patricia, Helen, and Robert. *Front row*: Dr. Ferguson, David, Sheelagh, Mrs. Helen Ferguson.

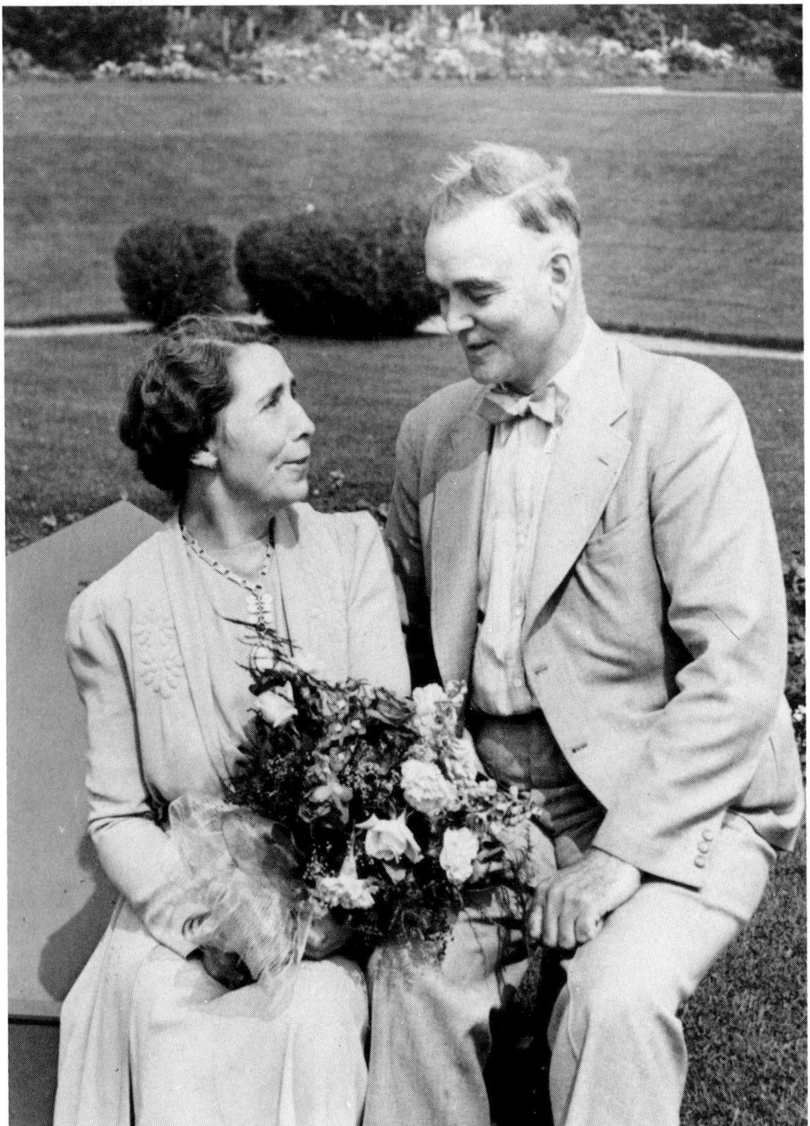

Courtesy of the Saskatchewan Lung Association

George and Helen Ferguson, 24 July 1942,
twenty-fifth anniversary of their arrival at Fort Qu'Appelle.

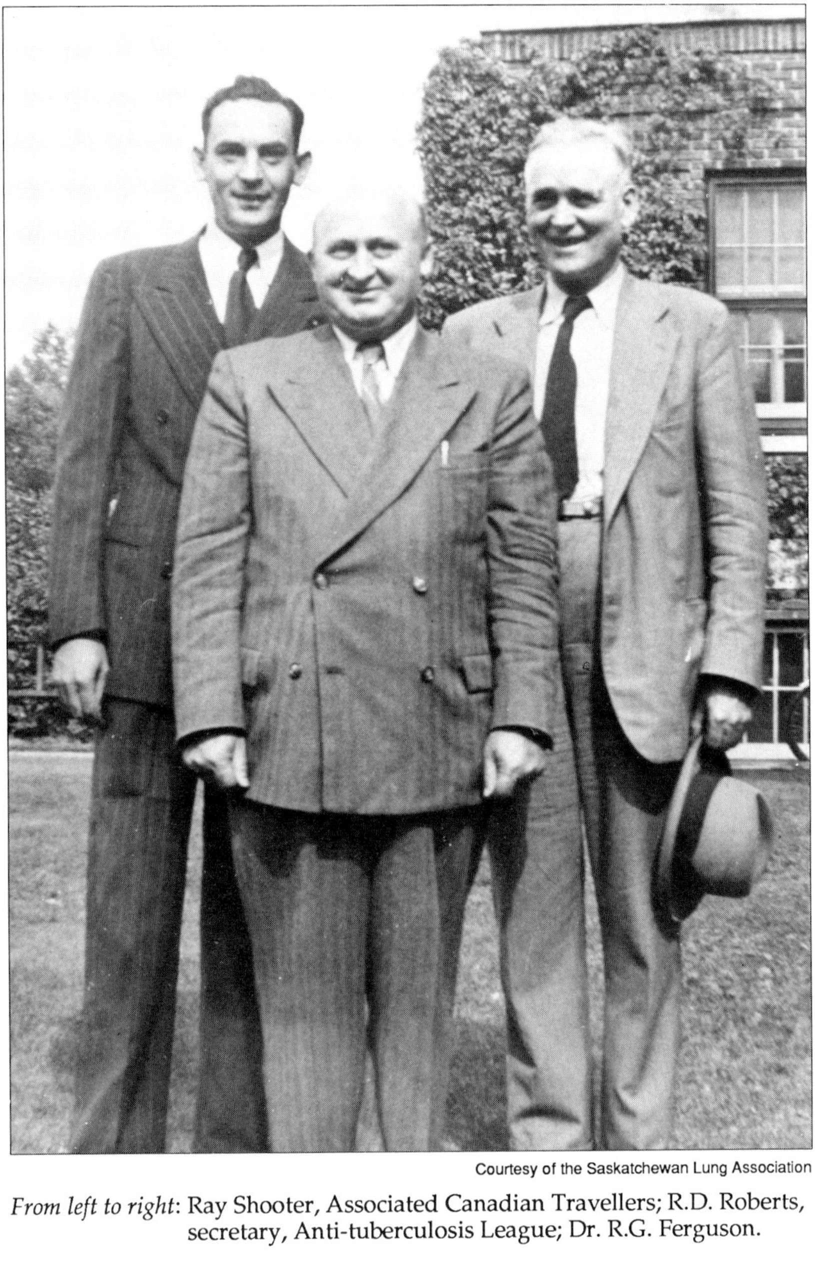

Courtesy of the Saskatchewan Lung Association

From left to right: Ray Shooter, Associated Canadian Travellers; R.D. Roberts, secretary, Anti-tuberculosis League; Dr. R.G. Ferguson.

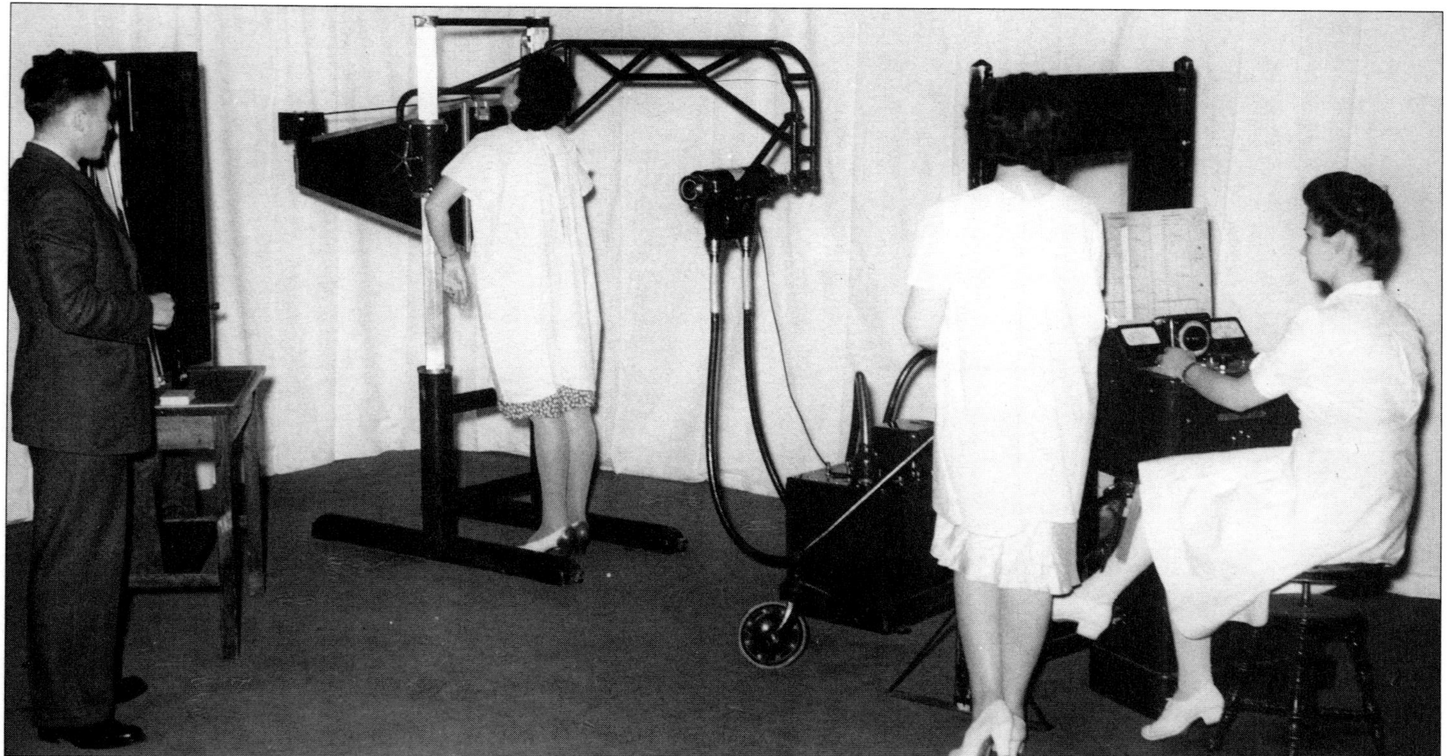

Courtesy of the Saskatchewan Lung Association

Robert Connell's home-made photofluorographic unit, 10 October 1941.
Perfectly counterbalanced by welder Richard Tizley, the machine moved up and down rapidly with fingertip control.

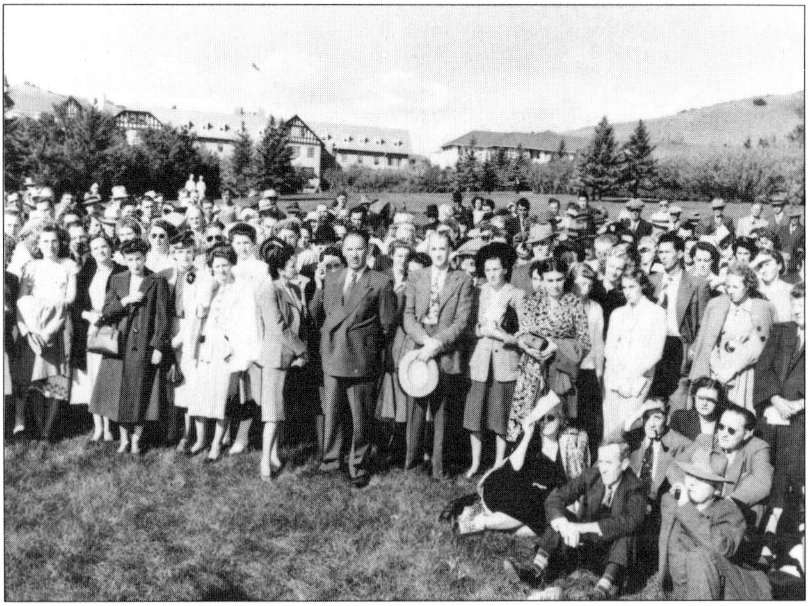

Courtesy of the Saskatchewan Lung Association

Ferguson's retirement, sixty-fifth birthday, 12 September 1948.

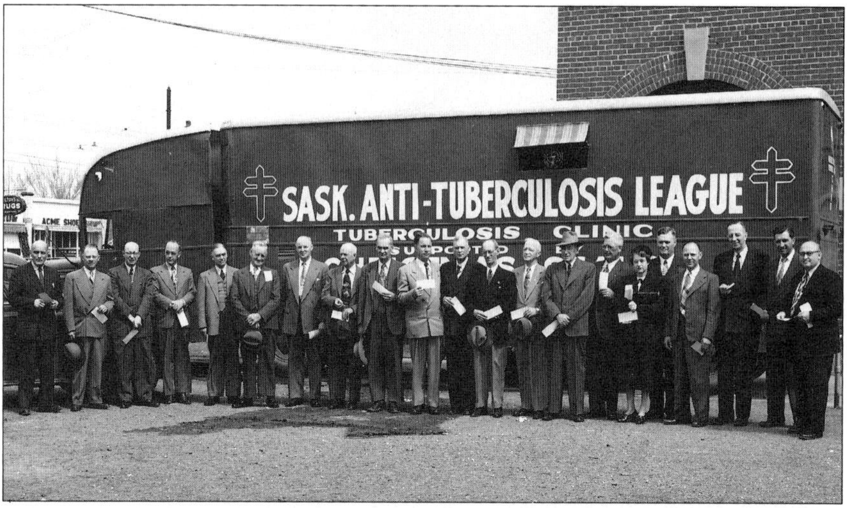

Courtesy of the Saskatchewan Lung Association

Photofluorographic Survey van and League directors (Ferguson is fifth from left), 1950.

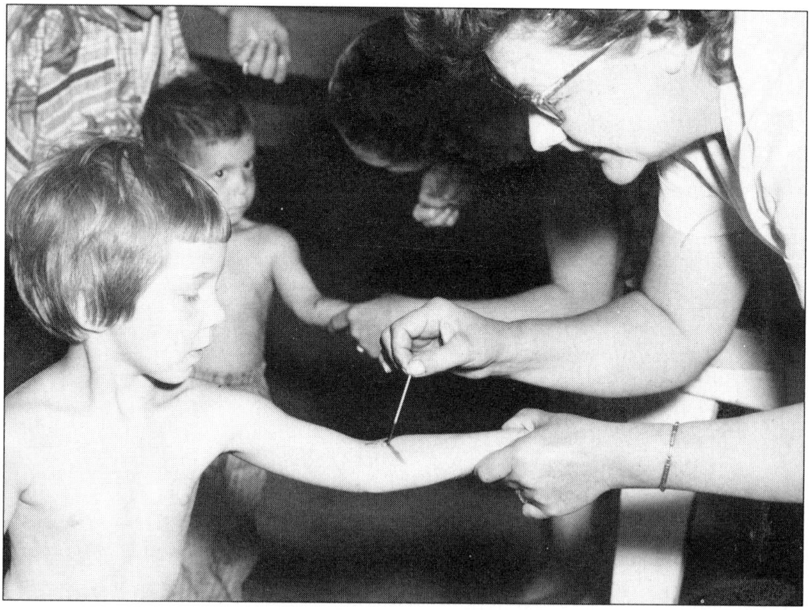

Courtesy of the Saskatchewan Lung Association

Tuberculin testing in 1960s.

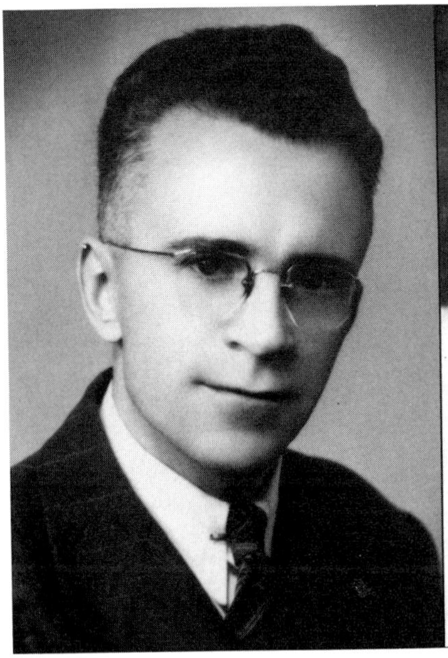

Courtesy of Mrs. Connell

Bob Connell.

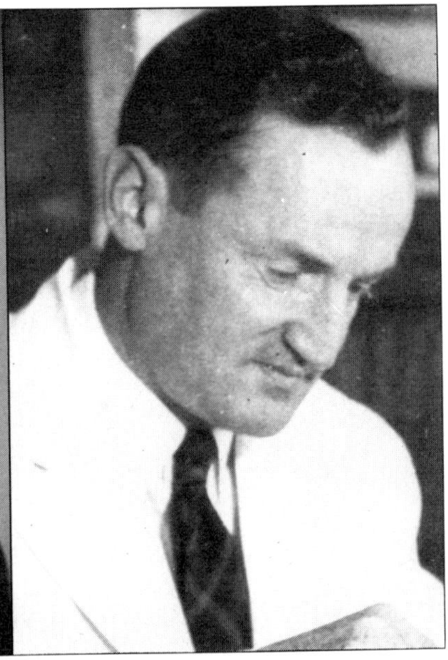

Courtesy of the Saskatchewan Lung Association

Dr. Thomas Wilfred Hamilton
(29 August 1894 – 3 September 1946).

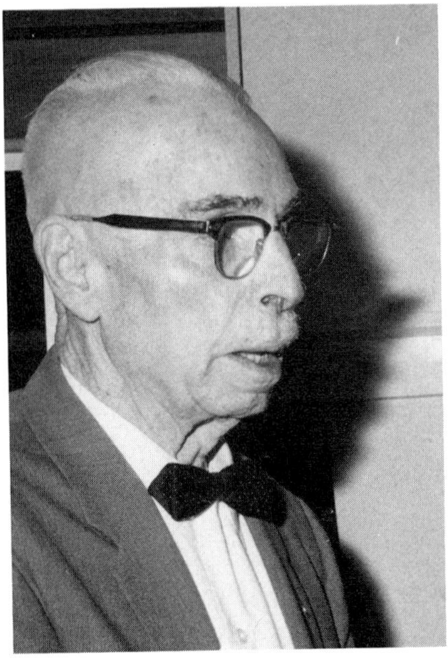

Courtesy of the Saskatchewan Lung Association

Dr. Robert Wellesley Kirkby
(12 September 1895 – 24 October 1976).

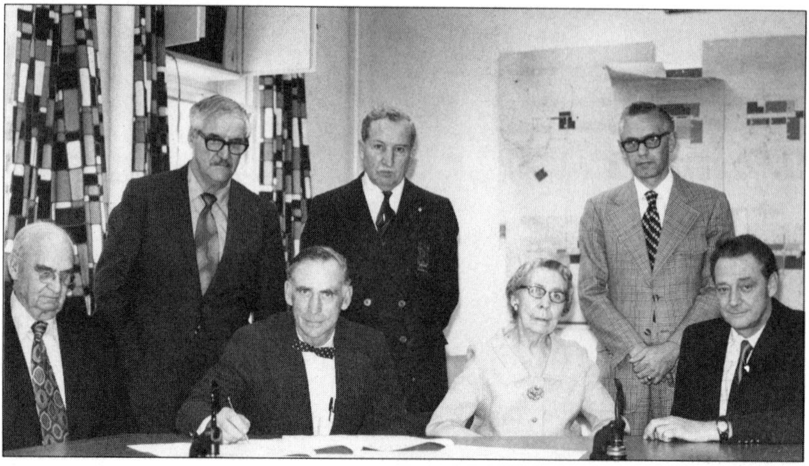

Courtesy of the Saskatchewan Lung Association

Ceremony to inaugurate Ferguson Professorship, University of Saskatchewan, 14 June 1973. *Back row*: Ken More, Saskatchewan Anti-tuberculosis League; J.W.T. Spinks, president, University of Saskatchewan; Earl Dick, executive-director, University Hospital; *Front row*: W.H. Howes, League; Dr. Robert Ferguson (son); Mrs. Helen Ferguson (widow); Cliff Wright, chairman, University Hospital Board.

are told by their physicians of the cost of treatment decide that they are unable to pay the charges and fail to make application." Nor was red tape ever interposed in any way between the sanatoria and any patient needing diagnosis or treatment.

Few could afford to pay for a year or more of treatment in a sanatorium. But, from 1917 until 1928, it was Saskatchewan's policy that "all who were able to pay were required to pay." In 1924, 29 of 295 patients (9.8 percent) paid part of the costs for their treatment, even though some were bankrupted and returned home penniless. By 1928, only 2.5 percent could pay for their treatment. The other 97.5 percent required at least partial financial help from their urban or rural municipal government.

Saskatchewan's Rural Municipal Act of 1920 required each rural municipality to contribute $100 annually to the sanatorium. In 1921, the $30,100 from 301 rural municipalities was set aside as the nucleus of a pool to pay for the treatment of indigent patients. Rural municipalities in this way got a head start on their urban counterparts, on the path to "free treatment."

The Saskatchewan Association of Rural Municipalities (SARM), at its annual meeting in March 1921, complained that the urban municipalities were exempt from this levy. In 1925, an urban pool was formed. Without such rural and urban contributions, the sanatorium would have been insolvent.

The first resolution to advocate totally free treatment for tuberculosis was introduced at the SARM annual meeting in 1925 by Ray Hart and Frank Freeman, reeve and secretary of the municipality of Bushville (Ray was the brother of Hazel Hart, who was then a patient in the sanatorium and who later edited the *Valley Echo*). Only six affirmative votes were cast that year among a meeting of 600 representatives. Yet the seed had been planted and the idea grew. In 1926, when the SARM had secured five directors on the League board for the first time, there were twenty votes in favour. In 1927 a different motion, that the provincial government take over direct control of the sanatoria, carried by a small majority. The government, normally very responsive to resolutions from SARM, countered that such an act would cause a diminution in support from many volunteer organizations.

At the annual meeting of SARM in March 1928, a momentous resolution was moved by Rural Municipality sixty-seven, Weyburn:

WHEREAS less than 10% of the patients treated in the Sanatoria operated by the Saskatchewan Anti-tuberculosis League are in a position to pay for the costs of their care and treatment thus leaving over 90% a direct charge on the public,
THEREFORE BE IT RESOLVED that we petition our Legislators to amend the Sanatoria Act so that all classes of T.B. patients shall have free treatment available at the public expense,
AND FURTHER that same be paid

a. partly by the Government
b. partly by all rural and urban municipalities in the province.

AND IT IS FURTHER SUGGESTED that the share of responsibility be apportioned as follows:
The Government to undertake all capital expenditure required in furnishing the necessary Sanatoria with their equipment and also contribute towards expense of care and treatment $1.00 per hospital day and the balance of care and treatment costs to be paid semi-annually by all municipalities of our province on an equitable basis.

In the midst of the discussion, an ex-patient of Fort Qu'Appelle Sanatorium, now cured and employed as secretary of his municipality for nine years, stood up. There, before the eyes of all doubting Thomases, it was remarked later, stood a living example of what could be and was being done through efficient and timely treatment of the tuberculous. This time the motion passed unanimously. A similar resolution was later passed by the Saskatchewan Urban Municipal Association and by the United Farmers.

Times were good just before the stock market crash and the Depression. The Liberal government of James G. Gardiner presented the Saskatchewan Sanatoria and Hospitals Act to the legislature before the end of 1928. This act provided for the cost of investigation of persons suspected of having tuberculosis and for their treatment. To ease the burden on the municipalities, exactly as the 1928 SARM resolution had requested, the government contracted to pay all capital expenses and to double its per diem payment for each patient in a sanatorium from fifty cents to one dollar. The government had already assumed ownership of the sanatorium buildings in 1923. When the new system of free treatment came into effect on 1 January 1929, the Rural Municipal Sanatorium Pool was disbanded. The Hon. Sam J. Latta, Minister of Municipal

Affairs, characterized the new act as "a great social experiment – and a costly one at that."

In his 1929 report, Ferguson cited numerous immediate benefits from free tuberculosis treatment:

> First, there was a gathering in of the hopeless sick from their homes to institutions . . . 296 additional active cases were removed from their homes . . . The effect of removing the financial barrier is earlier treatment, earlier isolation, and an increase in the number of days treatment and the gross cost, but the end result will be more cures and a shorter period of disability, lessened spread of the disease, a lower death rate, and eventually less new cases.

Some modification of the financial arrangements became necessary at once. For the first year of "free treatment," the rural levy, from 69 percent of the population, produced $264,688 or 81.2 percent of the total, while the villages, towns and cities paid only $61,418 or 18.8 percent. The act was amended in 1930; thereafter the rural municipalities paid 60 percent and the urban municipalities 40 percent. This arrangement seemed equitable until 1952, when levies came to be based one-third on the basis of population, one-third on total equalized assessments of property, and one-third on the number of treatment days. The municipal levy continued until 1979, thirty-two years after the advent of "free hospitalization" in Saskatchewan, and provided the League with a secure source of income not subject to the annual legislative budget process. More money came from municipal than from provincial coffers; in a year of restraint an individual municipality might spend as much on tuberculosis as on roads.

In 1931 a private member's bill sought to eliminate the "free" clause from the act but received no support from either the government or the opposition. The Hon. J.M. Uhrich, the former minister of health, thundered: "Let our fight be against tuberculosis, but never against the tuberculous."

The free enterprise concept of "user pay" was simply not practical or realistic for tuberculosis. Since most patients could not afford to pay for prolonged treatment, since local governments usually had to pick up the bill and since the stigma of accepting charity delayed people from coming for treatment, free treatment was a good example of a logical solution reached by members of a practical, cooperating, agrarian society. The benefits of free treatment were expressed in the increasing numbers of patients who presented early in the disease, the proportion rising from 14.3 percent of admissions in 1928 to 26 percent after two years and 43 percent after six years.

Elsewhere in Canada, universal free treatment was not adopted for years. Alberta, in 1936, became the second province to offer it, followed by Manitoba in 1944 and New Brunswick and Nova Scotia in 1946. Ontario assumed costs for indigents on 1 July 1938. Other provinces paid only for indigents and special groups until free treatment was phased in as a condition of the federal health grants to the provinces in 1948.

David A. Stewart, praising Saskatchewan's forward step in 1935, said, "We would never have eradicated smallpox if a man had had to mortgage his farm to pay for the treatment." Saskatchewan's health minister, Allan Blakeney, said in 1964, "The introduction of diagnosis and treatment of tuberculosis at public expense was one of the early and essential steps in developing a program of health services available to all." To have Saskatchewan lead all other jurisdictions in North America, the first to provide free treatment of tuberculosis, was one of Ferguson's greatest accomplishments.

The Depression, 1930–1939

Ferguson was no stranger to adversity but the financial difficulties of the Depression tested his mettle. His annual report in August 1931 testified to the threat to the League.

> In this, the year of the depression with its losses and financial embarrassment for those working for themselves and unemployment worries for those who work for hire, and lowered standards of living in the province generally, the responsibility resting upon the Saskatchewan Anti-tuberculosis League is perhaps the greatest since its formation. Financial difficulties – worry and lowered standards of living – are factors which predispose to tuberculosis, and present conditions have created all the greater need for anti-tuberculosis work and especially for the immediate care of the sick. Notwithstanding financial conditions, the sick require, and their friends expect, everything possible to be done that will restore them to health and useful employment at the earliest possible date. On the other hand the

> same financial conditions have given rise to the urgent need for retrenchment in order to lighten the burden of the taxpayer . . . The League must scrutinize every division of its organization in order to meet financial conditions.
>
> During the past year, a Committee of the Board have carefully gone into the detail of the administration of the various Sanatoria with a view to initiating economies. Later on the Secretary of the Department of Hospital Service of the Canadian Medical Association spent several days with us going over the details and methods of our Organization with a view to furthering efficiency. Recently . . . I had the opportunity of visiting several Sanatoria in the East, and of studying their methods with a view to increasing efficiency and economy . . . Only an early diagnosis and the most efficient treatment will restore the patient in the shortest number of days and send him home to employment at the least total cost. Less than efficiency prolongs treatment and is wasteful and costly.
>
> At the onset of 1930 the League was caught carrying a peak load of patients. Financial conditions were serious, and things looked bad, but as the year advanced there developed a turn for the better. First, there was a slight reduction of patients from March to the end of 1930. Also there was the reduction of per diem cost from the estimate of $3.04 to $2.92 in 1930 . . . Salaries will be lower, although we cannot expect too much in this direction. Owing to the fact that many of our employees are in contact with an infectious disease we can neither work them too hard nor can we reduce their standard of living . . . Tuberculosis is still the most serious infectious disease with which society has to cope today.

At the depth of the Depression Ferguson stood up at the New Year's banquet in 1932 to announce that the League was desperately short of funds. It had only two choices. Either a percentage of the staff would be discharged, or each member would have to take a proportionate cut in pay. Ferguson announced the extent of his own cut, 18.75 percent, the largest imposed on anyone in the system, and then the group assented to a smaller cut. At the end of this painful process, it is reported, he received "resounding applause." What other administrator would have been applauded for announcing a cut in pay? Saskatchewan government employees did not suffer their pay cut until six months later.

Ferguson's first salary reduction, from $8,000 to $6,500, dated back to October 1931; the next, 5 percent in March 1933, dropped his earnings to $6,175.20; and the third, in March 1935, to $5,961.60. At the same time his medical superintendents, Hamilton, Kirkby and Boughton, took only the first two cuts, from $5,000 to $4,500 in October 1931, and then to $4,322.40 in March 1933. Doctors Molony and McPherson each took a 5 percent reduction, while the other members of the medical staff were not subjected to any step of the belt-tightening exercise. Ferguson was anxious to keep a starting salary which would attract able doctors.

On one occasion during the Depression the League was unable to provide four married orderlies with the raise in salary they needed. Ferguson reported to these men that he was able to get a $5 monthly increase for each of them – but it came from his own pocket.

Wherrett later observed that Ferguson had been able to maintain and extend services during the thirties "only because the financial institutions, municipalities and the Provincial Government had complete confidence in both his ability and his integrity."

Preventorium

No matter how tight the money, the most cost-ineffective part of the operation, the Preventorium, continued in operation. Few other sanatoria could afford such a facility, but as a flagship operation, it epitomized prevention and thus was dear to Ferguson's heart. The Preventorium was built and its day-to-day operation largely financed by the IODE. Its first occupant, William Didorak, had been born outside the sanatorium in 1926. The first infant born in the delivery room, 6 April 1927, was named Merlin Ferguson Stewart. All, of necessity, received artificial feedings. The staff wasn't busy – on average there were only four infants in the Preventorium, each staying a year or so. The last infant cared for was Vernon Wayne Okemau, born on 16 August 1956.

Because exposure to the tubercle bacillus was prevented from birth, and the infants were vaccinated with BCG against the day when they would return home to their mother, all but one of these 210 infants (175 born in the sanatorium) went through childhood free from tuberculosis.

Introduction of Surgery

In spite of the stringent times which made the purchase of new equipment difficult, the medical staff began to use new interventionist treatments to collapse the lung, thus resting the most diseased lung to add to the bodily rest advocated for the entire patient.

With the acquisition of a fluoroscope it became possible to give pneumothorax treatments. Air was injected into the pleural space every one to three weeks, the degree of collapse being monitored with the x-ray fluoroscope. Pneumothorax was used sparingly at Fort San from 1920 to 1924, but sixty-seven patients received pneumothorax treatments in 1927.

Elsewhere, surgeons felt the ideal was a permanent lung collapse. To achieve this the first thoracoplasty at Fort San was performed in December 1925. With removal of upper ribs, much blood was lost, resulting in a rather high mortality and considerable disfigurement of the patient. Thoracoplasty did not become as popular in Saskatchewan as in Montreal, where chest surgeons, especially Norman Bethune and Edward Archibald, were enthusiastic and skilful in its performance.

Crushing the phrenic nerve was easier; by paralyzing the diaphragm it rested the lung on the same side. The first operation of this type was done in January 1929 by Dr. W.S. Barclay.

When an adhesion kept the lung tethered to the chest wall and prevented its collapse after the induction of pneumothorax, the adhesion was cut using a thoracoscope. The first operation of this type, pneumolysis, was done at Fort San in 1933.

Bronchoscopy, whereby a rigid tube with a light is passed through the mouth and trachea into the bronchi to observe disease directly, to collect pus for bacterial examination, and to biopsy abnormal lesions, arrived late at Fort San. The first bronchoscopy was carried out in the summer of 1936.

An interesting comparison between the results of veterans' treatment at Fort San and at the Central Alberta Sanatorium in Calgary was the topic of a 1984 University of Calgary history thesis by Darlene J. Zdunich, "Tuberculosis and World War One Veterans." Dr. A.H. Baker's staff at the Alberta institution performed over four times as many pneumothoraces as Ferguson's staff at Fort San. Barely half of the ex-soldiers who received pneumothorax in Alberta left the sanatorium alive and less than one-third improved. Although veterans admitted to Fort San had less favourable admission diagnoses, they were released with more hopeful discharge diagnoses. Zdunich concluded that the veterans at Fort San benefited from Ferguson's more conservative approach.

Fund-raising by Associated Canadian Travellers

Legend has it that at the worst moment of a cruel winter blizzard in 1934, Ferguson's automobile became stuck in the snow. He trudged to the somewhat obscured lights of the next railroad station and walked into the warm cheer of a railroad car. The occupants were travelling salesmen. During a long discussion, Ferguson explained the sorry plight faced by the sanatoria. He made such a deep impression that the travellers, newly organized as the Associated Canadian Travellers (ACT) and looking for a public service project, offered their assistance in the annual Christmas Seal campaign. Eiler's Jewelry of Regina stimulated further interest by offering the Eiler Trophy to the ACT club that raised the most money per member.

On another occasion Ferguson turned a winter calamity into good fortune. This time Bill Hart of Prince Albert's radio station CKBI was one of a group of travellers snowbound with Ferguson in Nipawin. Hart offered to sponsor a dance, with the music broadcast over his station. The listening audience could bring back their favourite performer to the microphone by phoning in to pledge a donation. The first performance was held at Parkside, forty miles west of Prince Albert, in January 1939. In spite of a snowstorm which forced the radio staff to use a railway jigger to get to Parkside, they raised $50. Soon the ACT added "amateur hour" broadcasts over CHAB Moose Jaw, CJNB North Battleford, CKRM Regina, CFQC Saskatoon, CKSW Swift Current and CJGX Yorkton. Yorkton won the Eiler trophy twenty times.

What a boon this was! The extra money allowed an extension of preventive services, especially clinics and surveys. Between 1934 and the end of 1955, the ACT raised $813,811 – and the Association of Rural Municipal Secretary-Treasurers raised another $58,000.

Economics

In 1933 Ferguson responded to a request from the Saskatchewan Registered Nurses Association for postgraduate instruction for unemployed nurses. To make this possible, the nurses volunteered that the stipends during such training be reduced from $35 to $25 per month. An extra class for postgraduate instruction was then arranged to assist ten additional nurses beyond the forty-two who had received instruction that year.

The economy deteriorated. Owing to continued crop failure, at its very worst in 1937, payments from the municipalities to the League fell far behind – by $160,189 in 1937 and another $143,137 in 1938. By the end of 1938, the total levies outstanding had reached $911,661; the League was forced to increase its borrowings to $671,082 and to pay $31,923 in annual interest. Saskatchewan nevertheless persevered with free treatment, rendered even more necessary by the Depression. At his retirement, Ferguson acknowledged that "the generous support from often limited funds was something that couldn't have happened in any other province." When the farm economy improved with good crops in 1939, muncipalities began to pay their overdue levies and indebtedness decreased. The Depression was over – but World War II brought its own problems.

— Chapter Six —

Tuberculosis Among Indians

PULMONARY TUBERCULOSIS IS perhaps the greatest curse the white man has inflicted upon the North American Indian. In 1815, Dr. Benjamin Rush from Philadelphia claimed "the consumption" was "unknown among the Indians of North America." His claim was accepted for years and appears to have been well-founded, except for the discovery of bone tuberculosis among disinterred collections of skeletons from Ontario, some of which predate the coming of the white man. Pulmonary tuberculosis and scrofula (lymph node tuberculosis) were found among the Sioux Indians of the Dakotas between 1835 and 1846, but the disease might already have been transmitted from white men farther east. Dr. James Walker, an Indian Agency physician in South Dakota, claimed that tuberculosis was present, but rare, among these widely dispersed nomadic peoples before the coming of the white man.

Ferguson reviewed the pertinent writings of the explorers (he listed ninety-five books he had read), interviewed surviving Mounties and traders, collected all available data, and held detailed discussions with Dr. William Hall, who had treated Indians continuously at Fort Qu'Appelle from 1882, and with Dr. Maurice M. Seymour, who had treated them from 1885 to 1904. Although Ferguson's sample size was rather small, the records for the nearby reserves allowed him to calculate rough mortality figures which have been quoted extensively ever since. Ferguson's inescapable conclusion was that Indians had greater susceptibility to some of the white man's diseases, particularly tuberculosis. In addition to tuberculosis, he reported epidemics of pertussis in 1887, of influenza and measles in 1890, of measles in 1898, and influenza in 1918–19, all of which caused further deaths. Each of his sources confirmed that, if there had been any cases of pulmonary tuberculosis among the widely scattered Plains Indians before the disappearance of the buffalo (about 1878) and the arrival of the white settlers, they were only sporadic.

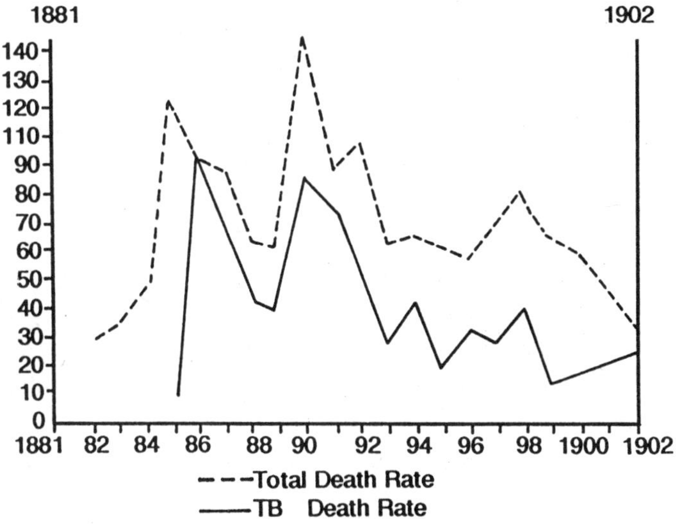

(Redrawn from Ferguson, R.G., Trans. Nat. Assoc. Prev. Tuberculosis *14*:5–56, 1928)

Figure 1: A tuberculosis epidemic among Red Indians of the Canadian Plains, 1881–1902. Annual death rate per thousand Indians.

Ferguson graphed the rapid increase in deaths from tuberculosis among the Indians at the Qu'Appelle and File Hills Agencies (Figure 1) as they settled in small houses in close proximity to each other on reserves. Under the new conditions of a stationary life, intermittent hunger and cultural demoralization, the annual Indian death rate from tuberculosis, roughly 1,000 per 100,000 population in 1881, quickly increased to reach the proportions of a serious epidemic by 1884, and became maximal in 1886. Deaths from tuberculosis peaked at 9,000 per 100,000 per year, about double the birthrate, and at the time accounted for two-thirds of all Indian deaths. By 1895 the rate had dropped to 3,000, by 1901 to 2,000, and by 1907 was down again to 1,000 per 100,000. Ferguson observed that there had been insufficient change in living or sanitary conditions to explain the drop. He correctly postulated that the peak tuberculosis death rate represented the acute stage of an epidemic arriving for the first time in a susceptible population. The severity could be explained by the fact that all ages were susceptible; deaths occurred among children, parents and grandparents at the same time. The subsequent drop, without treatment, represented a natural phenomenon as more resistant individuals survived. Virtually all Indian children were "tuberculized"; by the age of eleven to fifteen, over 96 percent had a positive tuberculin test.

Indians were not legally a responsibility of the Saskatchewan Anti-tuberculosis League, a provincial organization, but of the Government of Canada. However, by an agreement with the federal government in 1924, forty beds for Indians were allocated as a means of paying off the capital advanced near the end of the war. Once the Prince Albert Sanatorium opened in 1929, there were adequate beds for Indians, both adults and children. When the new Indian Hospital in Fort Qu'Appelle opened in 1936, Fort San transferred their Indian patients there. (In contrast, the Ninette Sanatorium did not accept Indian patients; Manitoba Indians gained access to sanatorium treatment only in 1946 when the Clearwater Sanatorium opened in wartime United States air force buildings.)

Research on Nearby Indian Reserves

Canada's National Research Council (NRC) was formed during World War I to help mobilize the scientific and industrial resources throughout the Empire. Members were appointed by order-in-council on 29 November 1916. It had three goals: "to coordinate the Federal Government's scientific activities; to support and promote industrial research; and to assist in the development of scientists by supporting their research activities."

The first NRC budget, for 1917–18, was only $13,794, with initial research directed to chemistry, mining and metallurgy. As individual problems arose which seemed to warrant practical research, from flax, honey and cold storage to industrial fatigue, an associate committee was formed to deal with each topic. The eleventh associate committee, as NRC President Dr. H.M. Tory explained, was formed in response to "resolutions passed by live stock associations all over Canada," who asked for help to fight disastrous outbreaks of bovine tuberculosis. Not until the formation in 1938 of the Associate Committee on Medical Research, which absorbed tuberculosis within its mandate, was there an NRC committee to deal with research in human medicine.

The Associate Committee on Tuberculosis held its first two meetings in 1925 and named the Fort Qu'Appelle Sanatorium as one of five Canadian research centers. Ferguson was awarded his first research grant of $2,000 in 1925, the year NRC funding for all eleven associate committees totalled $106,214. Ferguson's grant was renewed annually for another twenty-two years, and was doubled when BCG research was added, even though total NRC funding dropped to a low of $121,732 when the depression was at its worst in 1932-33.

Field work under the NRC grant began on 28 June 1928 when Dr. Ferguson and Dr. Kirkby from the sanatorium, and Dr. Urban Gareau, a Regina pediatrician, accompanied by Dr. Austin Simes, a general practitioner at nearby Abernethy, conducted a thorough examination of all Indian children up to two years of age at the File Hills Reserve. Simes had conducted a baby clinic on the reserve since 1924. Then, in July, Dr. William Hall of Fort Qu'Appelle, assisted by Ferguson, Kirkby, Gareau and Dr. F.C. Middleton of the Department of Public Health, examined another sixty-seven Indian children, four years of age and under, at Asham's Point on the Qu'Appelle Indian Reserve. Such surveys became annual events on both reserves.

Indian children attending the Lebret and File Hills Indian schools were the first to receive close medical scrutiny. In 1926, most were well nourished and in good general condition. All 315 children were tuberculin tested; 92.2 percent of them were sensitive to 1/400 mg of old tuberculin. Chest radiographs revealed that 8 percent had active lesions and another 11.4 percent had evidence of healed tuberculous lesions. Physical examination demonstrated enlarged tuberculous lymph nodes in the neck in 7 percent, while 4.7 percent had healed scars of previous discharge from these areas. Only 1 percent had evidence of previous bone tuberculosis.

All possible manifestations of tuberculosis were seen among the Indians, including pulmonary and bone lesions and occasional meningitis, but TB of the lymph nodes was unusually common. In 1906, at the Qu'Appelle Industrial School, 40 of 205 Indian children had been operated on for tuberculous lymph nodes. Since 7 percent of the Indian cattle tested positive for tuberculosis, and since about one-third of white children with enlarged lymph nodes at that time had ingested tuberculous milk, the initial presumption was that many Indian children had bovine tuberculosis. However, sophisticated culture methods and typing of the bacteria showed that all bacilli from Indian lymph nodes were of the human type. Besides, Indians had only beef cattle and did not drink milk!

Some Indian children with tuberculous lymph nodes made a perfect recovery. One, Paul Acoose, became a noted marathon runner. The prevalence of tuberculous lymphadenitis among Indian children subsided quickly, from 19.5 percent in 1906 to 7.4 percent in 1921 and to less than 1 percent in 1932. Pulmonary tuberculosis decreased more slowly.

Ferguson recognized the need to determine the prevalence of tuberculosis in adult Indians as well. How was he to get them together for chest radiographs far from electrical sources? He had the brilliant inspiration to join the annual treaty party, when all natives congregated to receive treaty money of five dollars each. He persuaded the Victor X-ray Corporation of Winnipeg to supply a portable x-ray machine and the Delco Light Company of Regina to supply a portable generator. In the second week of July 1927, all this equipment accompanied the treaty party to the File Hills Reserve where full compliance was achieved and 130 adult Indians were x-rayed. Another thirty-five were x-rayed at the Pasqua Reserve.

Ferguson studied the changes in food, clothing, shelter and sanitation coincident with the abandonment of the Indians' nomadic lifestyle in favour of settlement on reserves. In 1928, he reported at a meeting in Great Britain:

> The moral and physical weakening of the Indian has to do with the introduction of the horse . . . firearms . . . liquor, the exchange of their fur tunics for the blanket, the exchange of the clothes necessary for warmth for alcohol, the extermination of the buffalo and the beaver, the concentrations upon reserves, the change of housing, the change of food, the exclusion of sun

> . . . by the clothing of the children; the compulsory concentration of children in schools, the change of occupation from hunting and warring to agricultural pursuits, and, on the mental side, the psychical depression of conquest by the whites, dependence on Government rations for food, visible ravages of white man's diseases, desertion by, or incompetency of, their Michi-Manitou and triumph of Kitchi-Manitou, and failure of even the white man's religion to protect them . . . The nudity of the Indian children in summer . . . was ended abruptly . . . The agents, in their zeal . . . instructed the parents to clothe their children. Thus for the first time in the history of the race the bountiful summer sun's rays were largely excluded . . . a lowering of resistance to disease developed.

To La Loche by Canoe

In 1927 Ferguson took part in a remarkable journey to investigate the health of the Indians of northern Saskatchewan, and to provide prophylactic immunization against smallpox and diphtheria. The party consisted of the Hon. J.M. Uhrich, minister of public health, Dr. M.M. Seymour, deputy minister of public health, Fred Hill, a public health technician, and Ferguson. The daughter of Dr. John A. Amyot, the deputy minister of health for Canada, journeyed with them as far as Île-à-la-Crosse.

The party left Regina by train on Monday evening, 15 August, and reached Big River, the end of the steel, the next evening in a cold, dismal rain. Near the end of Crooked Lake Dr. Seymour's new motor canoe struck a submerged log – and His Majesty's Mail was set adrift. On the nineteenth they rested at Green Lake. There "the sensation of the day was our evening dip, when our fair charge, Miss Amyot, swam the lake without the consent of her guardian." For the rest of their trip they were joined by Robert Urquhart, manager of the Hudson's Bay Company at Green Lake. By nightfall of the twenty-first they reached Beauval and on the twenty-third, Île-à-la-Crosse. Here a brand-new twenty-bed hospital had replaced the old mission hospital begun by the Grey Nuns in 1873. Frank Read, the manager of the Hudson's Bay store, accompanied them to Buffalo River Post (Buffalo Narrows) on the twenty-fifth, then to Dillon and finally La Loche four days later. Here they attended to the Hudson's Bay Company post manager's infant daughter, who had been ill for five days. They agreed to transport a Chipewyan boy with tuberculosis of the hip 400 miles south to the sanatorium, placating him with a bright red silk handkerchief, some dried apples, a knife and a stick to whittle. While they were at Île-à-la-Crosse on the return journey, Dr. Amyot, as had been arranged, flew in from Big River by airplane in one and a half hours to inspect the new hospital, a trip that had taken the boaters three days. The canoes returned to Big River on 11 September, once again in pouring rain, completing "a delightful journey through one of Canada's most romantic and attractive playgrounds." The journey had taken four weeks. Four doctors had seen at first hand the high prevalence of tuberculosis in one of the most inaccessible portions of Saskatchewan.

Appointment of Simes to Indian Health Unit

In 1929, the Indian Department, at the behind-the-scenes behest of Ferguson, no doubt with overt backing from his friend William Richard Motherwell, the influential federal minister of agriculture from 1921 to 1930, named Dr. Austin B. Simes as full-time medical superintendent of the new demonstration unit named the Qu'Appelle Indian Health Unit. Simes had earlier taken special training in tuberculosis in Britain and had been medical health officer of part of the nearby File Hills Indian Reserve for ten years. Before taking up his new post, Simes joined the staff of the Fort Qu'Appelle Sanatorium for a few months to update his training.

Ferguson described Simes as "capable, energetic, and interested in the work." With the full support of the National Research Council, the two of them were about to embark on a well-planned research project with BCG.

Since chest radiographs were crucial to diagnosis, Ferguson decided that their reports must be standardized. He arranged to read over 100 consecutive chest radiographs himself with Dr. Maurice F. McPhedran of the Phipps Institute of the University of Pennsylvania, a speaker at the Winnipeg meeting of the British Medical Association in June 1930.

The Indians near Fort Qu'Appelle probably enjoyed better health than those on the average reserve, since medical care was close at hand, augmented by the full-time field nurse who was added to the research project staff. Following concentrated efforts at diagnosis, isolation and treatment, the death rate from tuberculosis among this population had dropped by 1931 to 279 per 100,000, compared to 586 for Indians throughout Saskatchewan and 539 in adjacent Montana. Yet the Indian death rate remained more than ten times greater than in the white population. Recognizing the close association between tuberculosis, poverty and poor living conditions, both Ferguson and Simes for some years had set themselves a more general goal of raising the standard of living among the entire Indian population. In 1929 and 1930, thirty-nine new houses had been built on the Qu'Appelle Reserve and seventeen on the File Hills Reserve.

The two schools in the research area, File Hills and Qu'Appelle, received careful annual attention, with prompt isolation and treatment of children with active disease. Between 1936 and 1939 only four previously healthy pupils contracted tuberculosis on the nearby reserves, as determined by a complete radiographic re-survey. The percentage of tuberculin-positive Indian children at the File Hills school declined from 92 percent in 1926 to 65.5 percent in 1937. In 1933 clinical and x-ray surveys of 800 children in eight more distant Indian residential schools revealed fifty (6.0 percent) with active tuberculosis, a much higher rate than in the Research Area.

Canada's record in dealing with tuberculosis among Indians had never been good. At its meeting in Ottawa on 7 December 1938 the executive of the Canadian Tuberculosis Association (on which Ferguson was the Saskatchewan representative) was informed of the gravity of the situation. Each year there were many more deaths from tuberculosis among Indians than there were Indians under treatment (805 deaths compared to 386 Indians under treatment). Saskatchewan's record in 1937 was the best of all the provinces, with about as many native patients under treatment as there were native deaths.

The Indian Advisory Committee met with the Hon. T.A. Crerar, minister of mines and resources, the cabinet minister with responsibility for Indians, and with officials of his Indian Affairs Branch. The committee pleaded for more treatment beds, for a demonstration project to provide supervision and segregation on the reserves, and for radiographic surveys. It strongly stated that such programs go hand in hand with health education and an attempt to improve living conditions on the reserves.

Northern Reserves

On 7 March 1933 the first aerial visit to a northern Indian community for a tuberculosis survey was undertaken. Dr. C.H. Andrews from the Prince Albert Sanatorium was flown from Prince Albert to Île-à-la-Crosse by Bill Windrum, a well-known bush pilot who made the trip under difficult conditions with his ski-equipped plane every two weeks. At night, the oil was drained from the engine and kept warm indoors. Before the warm oil was added the next morning the engine had to be heated with a blow torch under a tarpaulin.

Andrews examined fifteen patients at the Île-à-la-Crosse hospital, operated by the Grey Nuns, with Dr. E.P. Lavoie and Miss Rapetta, RN, in charge. Arrangements were made for a ten-year-old boy to be sent to Prince Albert Sanatorium on the next plane two weeks later.

Aerial trips soon became commonplace. For example, in 1937 Dr. Simes and Robert Connell flew to Lac la Ronge and Beauval to survey Indian schools, carrying with them a gasoline-driven generator. At the same time, Dr. Kirkby travelled regularly by road to Indians at the Duck Lake, Onion Lake and Delmas schools.

Day schools at Mistawasis, New Reserve, Sandy Lake, Sturgeon Lake, Little Pine, John Smith, James Smith, Beardy's, One Arrow, Okemasis, Cote and Keys had a higher rate of tuberculosis than those under closer scrutiny near Fort Qu'Appelle. In the study of these more remote schools in the fall of 1940, seventeen new cases of active tuberculosis requiring hospitalization were discovered among a group of 585 students (2.9 percent). Another forty-two cases of minimal tuberculosis required observation. Churches meant well when they set up residential schools, but it seems probable that the congregation of Indian children in such close proximity caused tuberculosis to spread more readily. In the north the epidemic ran its course later, because there the Indians had kept to their nomadic, uncrowded lifestyle for a generation longer than those in the south.

Ferguson declared that the greatest tribute bestowed on him during his active years of practice was given to him by the Indians. In 1935, the Qu'Appelle Valley Indians of the Muscowpetung, Piapot and Pasqua bands named him Chief Muskeke-O-Kemacan at a ceremony in his honour.

Vaccination with BCG

The Université de Montréal spearheaded research into BCG (bacillus Calmette-Guérin) vaccine in Canada. Production and experimental use of the vaccine in Montreal began in 1925. The next year, aided by the first of a series of $2,000 annual NRC grants, oral BCG vaccination was given to seventy-four newborn infants in Montreal, only two years after Calmette began the wide use of BCG in France.

Ferguson recognized Indians as the Saskatchewan group most likely to benefit from BCG. Compared to whites, Indians in 1926 were ten times more likely to die from TB. In Ferguson's eyes this justified the slight risk which might be present from the use of BCG. As an anonymous history in the NRC Archives states, this was "a highly controversial subject" which "occasionally resulted in acrimonious discussions," although Ferguson's studies, in which Dr. A.B. Simes collaborated, "were carefully laid out by members of the [NRC] statistical staff and the results were analyzed by them." In 1931, the NRC Associate Committee on Tuberculosis received a favourable report from its subcommittee on BCG, and the next year Ferguson received approval to begin BCG vaccination of newborn infants in the Fort Qu'Appelle Health Unit; his annual grant was raised to $4,500, which represented a substantial share of the $28,900 allotted for tuberculosis research in Canada. To show his faith in the method, Ferguson vaccinated his own six children with BCG before embarking on his study.

In the BCG study families of comparable status in respect to housing, sanitation and certain other economic and social factors likely to affect the health of children were paired, and one family of each such pair was allotted at random to one of two groups, designated "Group A" and "Group B." All children born into the families of Group A were vaccinated in one year, while all children born into families of Group B in the same year were taken as controls. In the following year this situation would be reversed and so on throughout the study. Vaccination of every second infant, carefully matched, was crucial to the integrity of the results. Ferguson phoned Austin Simes at least once each week to get a list of the births and to ascertain whether the newly born infant was placed in the BCG group or the control group.

For the first twenty-one newborn infants, in 1933, BCG vaccine was administered in a teaspoon with a little lukewarm milk, half an hour before feeding, three times on alternate days for the first ten days of life. If the mother was known to have tuberculosis the infant was kept separate from the mother for six weeks until some immunity could develop. Beginning in 1934, BCG was administered intracutaneously, the initial dose of 0.3 mg being soon reduced to 0.2 mg. Oral revaccination was performed at one and three years of age, again in three doses at forty-eight-hour intervals.

Covering letters from Dr. Armand Frappier at the Faculté de Médicine, Université de Montréal, show that each batch of BCG vaccine had been tested aerobically and anaerobically, and that the "200 guinea pigs vaccinated since last January" were "feeling better and better" as "witness to the purity of the strain."

Between 1933 and 1943, 306 Indian infants were vaccinated at birth and another 303 served as controls. Each child was tuberculin tested and examined annually. Whenever a tuberculin reaction was negative, revaccination was carried out at three-year intervals. By 1947 the incidence of tuberculosis was nearly five times greater in the unvaccinated and the disease was more severe and more widely spread throughout the body than in the vaccinated group. Postmortem examinations were performed whenever possible and included 64 percent of the fatalities among the vaccinated group. There was no evidence whatever of any recurrence of virulence of the BCG strain in the vaccinated group, a theoretical possibility greatly feared by experts.

Because 5 percent of the nurses in Western Canadian hospitals "broke down" with tuberculosis, all tuberculin-negative student nurses in Saskatchewan hospitals and tuberculin-negative sanatorium and mental hospital employees were given BCG. This measure reduced the number of cases of manifest tuberculosis to less than a quarter of the previous rate for nurses and to one-fifth of the previous rate for sanatorium employees. In subsequent years, tuberculin-negative members of families in which tuberculosis had occurred were vaccinated, contacts of recent cases first and then families of all ex-patients.

Ferguson's BCG studies were made in the face of frank hostility to BCG throughout the English-speaking world, especially in the United States. As D.J.C. Phillipson wrote in 1983, "English-speaking North American researchers mistrusted live-bacteria vaccines." Ferguson had not proceeded rashly, however, since by the early 1930s one million had already been vaccinated elsewhere; 425,000 in France and 204,000 in French Indo-China. In addition to what Dr. Boughton called a "vague but deep-seated hostility" toward the use of BCG in the United States, there were some valid objections: BCG was not more than 80 percent effective, whereas smallpox vaccine was 100 percent effective; BCG suppresses a valuable instrument of diagnosis and epidemiological surveillance, since it causes a positive tuberculin reaction; by rendering the tuberculin reaction valueless, BCG eliminates the possibility of using chemoprophylaxis such as isonicotinic acid hydrazide (INH) for newly exposed individuals; the first use of BCG in France was conducted without properly controlled studies (though better studies soon appeared from Norway and Sweden), therefore the French studies could not be quoted to justify the use of BCG in Canada; there was a catastrophic rash of deaths in Lubeck, Germany, in 1930–31 from the use of a live and contaminated tuberculosis vaccine; there was a real but unfounded fear that the bacteria might regain their virulence; and vaccination by cutaneous injection often caused ulceration of the lymph nodes under the armpit, leaving a prominent scar. To make the scar less visible, nurses and other adults often chose to receive BCG into the skin over the upper thigh.

Today there has evolved one further objection to the use of BCG. People with reduced immunity, particularly those infected with the human immunodeficiency virus (HIV) of acquired immunodeficiency syndrome (AIDS) have weak, dying and dead white blood cells which lack the strength to imprison even a weakened BCG germ; the defending white blood cells may become overwhelmed by the attenuated bacilli of BCG, and death is possible in such immunodeficient persons.

When Ferguson died in 1964, Dr. Boughton paid tribute to his work with the BCG vaccine:

> No record of Dr. Ferguson's place in the history of Saskatchewan would be complete without reference to his introduction of the preventive vaccination against tuberculosis by B.C.G. (Bacillus Calmette Guérin). He had taken me with him to see the groundwork being done in Paris by the originating physicians at a time when it was scorned in Great Britain and hardly known in North America. Already, having an intimate knowledge of tuberculosis among the Qu'Appelle Indians, he saw at once the possibility of controlling their tuberculosis. However, in tuberculosis circles there was much questioning about the safety and the morality of introducing live tubercle into the human body . . . But his reasoning and his faith told him he was right so he vaccinated his own children. (I also vaccinated my children before vaccinating others.) Since there were no untoward results he introduced a B.C.G. vaccination program among the infants in the Qu'Appelle Indian Health Unit. Five years later infant deaths from tuberculosis were only 20% of what they had been. In recent years all Canadian Indian infants which can be reached are vaccinated with B.C.G. Then came the protection of sanatorium employees and the nurses in eight general hospitals. More recently the World Health Organization has initiated vaccination programs in the developing and underdeveloped countries.

Ferguson's long-term BCG research was supported financially by the National Research Council for twenty-three years. His studies ceased only when he retired. Armand Frappier has said that this was the first intensive and prolonged BCG study in the world to be supported officially.

If Simes had used the simplest of all randomizing methods, the flipping of a coin, the BCG study might have counted as the world's first truly randomized medical research study (except for studies such as those of James Lind who tried different scurvy remedies on small groups of men), antedating the penicillin studies in Britain in the early 1940s. Indeed, Ferguson and Simes, when they published their results in 1949, stated that theirs was a "randomized" study, and thus inferred that it was not simply a matter of giving BCG to alternate infants. Although Ferguson was usually careful in his choice of words, minutes of the NRC's Associate Committee on Tuberculosis for 17 June 1936 contain statements that negate any such claim: "It was found more convenient to vaccinate the children born in the hospital and for that reason the greater proportion of the controls had been born in the home." Nevertheless, the panel on tuberculosis of the NRC Associate Committee on Medical Research in 1946 felt Ferguson's study was "the most scientific trial of BCG yet made." The war history written by associate committees of the NRC gave credit to Ferguson's BCG study for "an experiment which is probably unique in the similarity of its experimental and control groups," praising the "unusual degree of medical control and the stable habits of the Indians" which made this possible.

Chapter Seven

The Last Decade

Photofluorographic Surveys, 1943–1947

SASKATCHEWAN LED THE world in mass radiographic surveys of an entire region, although selected groups in Brazil and Germany had participated in somewhat haphazard mass surveys. Ferguson dreamed of being able to detect virtually all patients with tuberculosis when the disease was in its early stages and most likely to be curable – and, he hoped, before the disease had been transmitted to others. But his dream required new technology, which might never have been realized if it had not been for the Connell brothers whose careers he had sponsored.

The story begins in early 1923, when Robert S. Connell was on staff as "assistant technician, x-ray" at a salary of $420 per year, ready to take over from Spencer Uren. Later, Robert's brother James was also hired. In addition to his apprenticeship at the sanatorium, James had gained experience with Dr. Clarence Millwood Henry, a Regina radiologist. The two Connell brothers had a natural talent for radiography. Robert pioneered the makeshift methods for taking a portable generator and x-ray machine to the File Hills Indian Reserve and to Indian schools for Dr. A.B. Simes. When the Prince Albert Sanatorium opened, James became its radiographer.

Chest radiographs offered a promising means for mass surveys but Christmas Seal funds were insufficient to purchase full-size fourteen-by-seventeen-inch film at ninety cents each for every Saskatchewan resident. Americans had experimented with a smaller four-by-five-inch film with considerable savings. Ferguson heard of the work of Manoel de Abreu in Brazil; by 1937 de Abreu was making 200 examinations per day in Rio de Janiero, using a 35 mm camera and roll film which reduced costs to about one cent per patient.

Was equipment available in Canada? Some experimental work was going on in several American centres but nothing suitable could be purchased. Ferguson assigned the project to Robert Connell. The most advanced "x-ray machines" of that time had a fluoroscope attached with which a radiologist could, for example, by observing the patient swallowing barium, examine the movement of the esophagus and stomach. Connell experimented with a new, faster fluorographic screen which gave a better image. Photofluorography involved a five-times higher radiation dose than standard radiography using a full-size film. The dose was increased even further by the longer film exposure of one-third of a second obtained while the fluoroscope was turned on for a full second at seventy kilovolts peak and six hundred milliamperes. The exposure time would have been even greater had not the distance between the x-ray tube and the fluoroscopic screen been reduced to thirty-six inches. The resultant greater magnification of the heart as compared to the usual seventy-two-inch distance of conventional chest radiography was less of a disadvantage in a sanatorium where the lungs were the focus of interest.

Another important development was the rotating anode tube which allowed a smaller focal spot and sharper definition of the image without excessive heat buildup on the anode. The interval between exposures was now determined by the time it took to place the next patient in position, and no longer by the need to allow the anode to cool. Connell mounted the camera rigidly on one end of a light-tight box, attached to an easily adjustable, counterbalanced stand (built by Richard Tizley, a welder hired by Ferguson on the day World War II began). The fluoroscopic screen was at the opposite end of the box and the entire box was lined with a thin sheet of lead to reduce scattered radiation. It was absolutely essential that the focal spot of the x-ray tube, the centre of the fluoroscopic screen, and the axis of the lens were perfectly aligned and that all vibration was eliminated. Slight movement anywhere in the system would cause a blurred image.

At first the miniature films were not of the highest quality, but they improved when Connell located a top-quality f1.5 German lens. Soon afterwards he found a physicist at Corning glass works in the United States, who, as a special favour, applied his experimental coating of fluoride to the lens in a vacuum, increasing its speed by another 75 percent. Then, by trial and error, Connell determined the best available film to use with the new equipment.

Similarly, Connell designed and built processing equipment with special film dryers. He devised an identification system and a card system to go with it. Ten to fifteen rolls of 35 mm movie-type film were developed simultaneously in a small fourteen-ounce tank. Dust and scratches, which would be greatly magnified on the processed film, were avoided. Developing, fixing, washing and drying took about two hours. Cost of film and processing was about one-fiftieth that of a standard radiograph. By 1947, 70 mm film was used to show abnormalities in greater detail. Later, the results were further improved by a photoelectric timing device which, by automatic control of milliamperage and time, reduced the radiation dose and virtually guaranteed uniform exposures.

An ancient second-hand van was purchased for $250; for another $400 it was converted into a mobile x-ray laboratory. Connell encountered new problems with every move, but by the summer of 1941 mobile photofluorography was ready. The trial run began at the Indian school at nearby Lebret, then moved on to Melville, Estevan and Regina; 7,982 individuals were examined. Although the equipment was usually moved into a building for a survey, the trailer had been fitted with a control panel and three dressing rooms so it could function independently.

Fifty to fifty-five images were taken on each roll, the film being advanced between each patient. Three to four people were radiographed each minute. By the second year 1,000 people could pass through during a seven-hour working day. Connell and his team established a record throughput of 2,455 people in one long day.

Detail was not as clear as that of a full-sized radiograph. About 10 percent of the abnormalities visible on a full-size chest radiograph were not recognizable on these miniature films. The more advanced the tuberculosis, the easier the detection. When an abnormality was suspected on the miniature film, a full-size fourteen-by-seventeen-inch film was obtained.

The sanatorium physician projected the films onto a ten-by-twelve-inch white matte screen for interpretation. G.D. Barnett tells how, during public surveys, Ferguson would read the 35 mm films in one corner of the village hall. He did this publicly, not privately, so when farmers and village residents gathered round, he would take the opportunity to teach them. He would also invite the local physician over to "help" him. The film strips were filed with 100,000 miniature chest films in an ordinary x-ray filing cabinet drawer.

Increased funds from Christmas Seal sales made it possible, even in wartime, to equip a second truck with a portable fluoroscope and camera. A third truck was purchased with $83,500 raised by Bill Shultz's program on radio station CHAB, though Shultz died before all the donations had been received. The combined length of the truck and trailer was 41 feet. The trailer itself was 28.5 feet long, 8 feet wide and 10 feet high, insulated, built of steel and lined with white enamel. The heavy generator was placed in the front of the trailer over the dual rear wheels of the truck. The examining room was 14-by-8 feet. There was also a built-in darkroom. During a survey, a canopy was raised between the trailer and an adjoining building which could then be used as a dressing room. If the truck had to be parked on sloping ground, it could be levelled with a jack. At first, each patient undressed and put on a hospital gown. Later, patients were radiographed in a shirt or blouse, provided it was not rayon and that all pockets were emptied. The new slogan became, "Keep your shirt on."

In 1942, Moose Jaw became the first city in North America to x-ray the chests of virtually all its residents. In addition, the inhabitants of eleven towns, four villages and fourteen rural municipalities were examined, a total of 42,663 people. Fifty-seven new, active cases of tuberculosis were discovered in addition to fourteen previous patients with reactivated disease.

Other preventive work for 1942 included 3,166 new patient referrals, 5,219 ex-patient recalls, 2,542 ex-patients examined by travelling consultants, and 233 contacts assessed by family doctors and examined with full-size radiographs. In addition, 1,233 children from Indian residential schools, twelve Indian reserves and three Indian day schools were examined as part of the NRC project. All this cost $45,540.53, only $578.73 more than had been raised in the Christmas Seal campaign.

In 1943, with the third unit now in operation, the photofluorographic survey examined 82,135 individuals. Seventy-six active cases of tuberculosis were detected. Viewing the survey "as a means for the discovery of unknown spreaders," Ferguson reported enthusiastically, "the gleam of hope for the eradication of tuberculosis has been fanned into a healthy blaze." Nevertheless, in that year Saskatchewan's tuberculosis deathrate rose to 29.8 per 100,000, well above the 24 per 100,000 level achieved in three years in the 1930s. Various wartime influences no doubt contributed to this increase.

In 1944, Ferguson reported that "extreme difficulties have been experienced throughout the year because of the rapid turnover and depletion of staff. Additional members of the staff have continued to join the forces as the call to duty became more urgent." However, the public responded with enthusiasm to the community surveys, turning out in large numbers and contributing a generous $95,000 to the Christmas Seal Fund. Most of the population of Regina and six other cities were examined, with 121,847 persons participating and another 3,721 involved in special studies. One hundred and five new patients with active tuberculosis were discovered.

Ferguson sent his persuasive organizer, R.D. Roberts, to secure the cooperation of an entire community, including its radio station and newspaper. In Regina Mrs. A.M. Walker enlisted 2,300 women volunteers, 800 of whom canvassed the city, house by house, with "request cards." Those who didn't wish to be x-rayed were contacted by staff from the Regina health department, who persuaded half of them to change their minds. A new appointment was issued to those who had failed to attend. Service clubs provided free transportation for the disabled. Five hundred volunteers staffed the office and the telephones. Ferguson told the observer from the Canadian Tuberculosis Association, "You learn something new from every survey."

In 1945, the survey employed university students as assistants. One unit began in Melville and worked west along the CNR main line. Another worked east from Balcarres and Lemberg towards the Manitoba boundary. They examined 138,936 individuals in rural areas and 1,491 university students and detected eighty-three new cases of tuberculosis.

By August 1947 the miniature x-ray survey of every city, town, village, rural municipality and local improvement district in Saskatchewan had been completed. It had reached 604,297 people or 74.1 percent of the non-Indian population. A program for the second-time-over was immediately launched; 74,892 were examined in the new campaign before the end of 1947.

Each community competed to surpass the achievement of other centres. In 1948, there was the highest-ever rate of participation (95.5 percent) in the Saskatoon survey when 41,082 residents were photofluorographed from an available population of 43,016. Ferguson was extremely gratified as he calculated that persons out-of-town, the sick, and those opposed on religious or other grounds made up close to 10 percent of the population. The enthusiasm and publicity generated by the Associated Canadian Travellers in their fund-raising drives ensured a higher turnout than was achieved in most other provinces in the years to follow. The cost efficiency was high due to the thousands of volunteers who contributed their time and effort.

Exposure to radiation was less of a concern than the threat from tuberculosis itself. At first, there was little or no shielding of the x-ray tube, and little effort to collimate, that is, to restrict the beam to the exact area of the film. Radiation was scattered to adjacent areas. It was not yet considered important to protect the technician with a lead apron.

In 1950, W.W. Van Allen, a physicist with the Division of Tuberculosis of the U.S. Public Health Service, monitored an American photofluorographic unit for five weeks. At the start of the check, 20 percent of the technicians received in excess of 300 mr (milliroentgens) per week, considered to be the upper limit of safety. After protective policies had been instituted, only 12 percent were exposed to more than 50 mr per week. (Thirty years later, few diagnostic x-ray technicians received more than 50 mr in an entire year.) By 1956, Dr. Edward Chamberlain, professor of radiology at Temple University, Philadelphia, reported that the gonadal dose could reach 25 mr from a miniature photofluorograph, compared to a much smaller dose from conventional radiography. His findings created consternation. The use of photofluorography decreased, in part to reduce the radiation dose, but also because of the greatly diminishing returns from mass surveys as fewer new cases of tuberculosis were uncovered each time. By 1961, Saskatchewan's surveyors carried out tuberculin tests on a first visit and two days later radiographed only those whose skin tests were positive. In 1966, with tuberculosis well controlled by chemotherapy, the Wherrett-Grzybowski report to the Saskatchewan government recommended the elimination of mass tuberculosis surveys and the gradual closing of sanatoria beds. By 1970, photofluorography was no longer in use.

Postwar

A 1943 Canada-wide survey of available tuberculosis beds showed that Ontario and Saskatchewan were far ahead of other provinces. Only Ontario, a wealthier province, and Saskatchewan had achieved the ideal ratio of three beds for every tuberculosis death. The rest of Canada, the survey concluded, required construction of 6,580 new sanatorium beds. Nevertheless, Fort San acquired the new West Wing, which opened in 1945 with accommodation for fifty adults, thirty-five children and the Preventorium. These were "replacement beds," the last to be built at any Saskatchewan sanatorium.

Table 2

RATIO OF TUBERCULOSIS DEATHS TO AVAILABLE TUBERCULOSIS BEDS

	Deaths per Year			Beds	Beds/Death
	White	Indian	Total	Present	Ratio
P.E.I.	66	1	67	87	1.3
Nova Scotia	420	9	429	681	1.6
New Brunswick	315	9	324	556	1.7
Quebec	2,609	44	2,653	3,576	1.3
Ontario	1,034	116	1,150	3,671	3.2
Manitoba	207	160	367	899	2.4
Saskatchewan	160	110	270	822	3.0
Alberta	150	162	312	409	1.3
B.C.	360	204	564	930	1.6

One of Ferguson's last initiatives was an eight-week affiliation course for each student nurse in Saskatchewan; it provided experience in tuberculosis and long-term illness nursing. Between 1 June 1945 and May 1964, 3,774 student nurses took the course at either Fort San or Saskatoon. Transportation expenses and sickness insurance were paid by the sanatoria. A twenty-six-week course for nurses' aides began at the Saskatoon Sanatorium in July 1947, a first for the province.

There was a high incidence of tuberculosis among patients in mental hospitals. At Ferguson's behest, tuberculosis patients were segregated from the others in 1936, placed in a separate fifty-bed unit in 1951, and finally moved to a new $400,000 tuberculosis wing under the charge of Dr. B. Kobrinski at Weyburn Provincial Hospital in June 1956.

As Ferguson reported, "The postwar era dawned with heartfelt gratitude and relief, and forthwith presented . . . new problems." By the end of 1945, World War II veterans occupied 150 TB beds. These included men whose disease had flared up during active service, and many more with minimal disease detected on a chest radiograph at the time of demobilization.

When Dr. Tommy Hamilton died in 1946, Dr. John Orr replaced him as the medical superintendent at Fort San.

The 1930s and the war years had seen many successes in Ferguson's campaign against tuberculosis. Now, the anticlimax of peace and national slackening of resolve brought frustration and disappointment.

Although Saskatoon had been ahead of Toronto in 1914 as the first city in the British Empire to forbid the sale of raw, uncertified milk and cream, Saskatchewan in other respects lagged far behind the rest of the provinces, notably Prince Edward Island, in the campaign against bovine tuberculosis. In spite of continued pressure from Ferguson, the federal Restricted Area Plan involved only six Saskatchewan municipalities in 1926 and another five in 1927. Cattle in the southwest ranching areas did not become tuberculosis-free until 1952.

In his 1945 report, Ferguson regretted he had "a small group of chronic convalescent cases for whom there is still no adequate provision. Some of them are up in years and have no homes to which to go, to complete convalescence. Some have received every treatment and are still infectious and unable to return to their homes. The Government has been requested by the League to build a pavilion at Fort Qu'Appelle especially equipped with a hobbycraft shop for occupational therapy and a rehabilitation department which will further assist this class of patients." This particular dream came close to fruition. The CCF (Co-operative Commonwealth Federation) government of Tommy Douglas was unusually sympathetic to health in general and to Ferguson and the fight against tuberculosis in particular. The government estimates for 1946 allowed for construction of a convalescent pavilion in 1947. However, Ferguson's final report, for 1947, observed, "We still lack accommodation for homeless cases who continue to be spreaders after receiving the maximum benefits of treatment . . . The construction of the convalescent pavilion, provided for in the 1946 estimates of the Government, has not been carried out owing to difficulties in securing building materials and skilled labour." This unit was never built, although the need for it had been apparent since 1931 when Dr. C.O. Banting, at Ferguson's request, reported on the need for a convalescent unit as a halfway house for "hardening up a patient and restoring his function under medical supervision." Manitoba, on the other hand, surged ahead of Saskatchewan in the provision of a rehabilitation program.

Almost every year, Ferguson pleaded with the Department of Indian Affairs to open a special "spreaders' school" for Indian children with minimal tuberculosis. He believed all tuberculous Indian schoolchildren in the province should be concentrated in one place to reduce contagion, and pressed this need upon Dr. H.W. McGill, director of the

Indian Affairs Branch of the federal Department of Mines and Resources, on 7 December 1938. But the federal government turned a deaf ear.

The election of the CCF government under T.C. Douglas on 15 June 1944 ushered in a new era in labour relations. Legislation fostered the formation of trade unions throughout the public sector. The possibility of confrontation with employees at the sanatorium, and the birth of the new viewpoint of "what can the San do for me?" instead of "What can I do to help the patients?" was not something Ferguson had foreseen. With almost daily skirmishes, new rules and new methods were worked out. Confrontation was not Ferguson's style, yet it became unavoidable. Ferguson had been accustomed to mutual respect between staff and management with everyone pitching in for the good of the institution and its patients. The sanatoria were operating under difficulties. Many of the orderlies, maintenance staff, nurses and some doctors had joined the war effort at home and abroad. Yet servicemen invalided home were arriving in increasing numbers, and a new dormitory was being erected at Fort San. It was all Ferguson could do to find a solution for each staffing problem as it arose.

Ferguson and his secretary, Frank Froh, would pick up the union president and take him to Regina for participation in tough negotiations. It was a new and very tiring experience for Ferguson. New legislation redressed traditional inequities and unfairness to employees; work hours decreased; wages increased. More staff were needed to do the same amount of work, yet, with the country still at war, it was impossible to recruit even up to prewar strength.

The "give and take" which formed the "great spirit" of the first twenty-eight years quickly evaporated. On occasion, an employee would quit work the minute the eight-hour day ended. Unemptied trays were set down. Beds were left unmade.

Ferguson aged noticeably and rapidly under these new conditions. In the evening, he would come home exhausted. After supper, he would go upstairs, listen to the news on the radio, and crawl into bed. Three years under the new regime were enough to wear him out.

Ferguson's Final Report

Ferguson's final annual report, in 1947, was memorable, for it gave expression to his philosophy, his goals and his lifetime achievement. These can be summarized as follows:

- Early diagnosis (empty beds were filled with newly discovered early cases).
- Improved treatment (surgery was still offered to those who presented late in their disease).
- Prevention (exposure of Saskatchewan children to tuberculosis had decreased greatly; the tuberculin-positive rate in children had dropped from 51 percent to 6 percent and in Normal School students from 76 percent to 17 percent).
- Protection of infants born to tuberculous mothers (this was, by 1927, achieved with the Preventorium).
- Research (he proudly listed the topics studied since 1922: early diagnosis; tuberculosis in families; tuberculosis among contacts, immigrants, schoolchildren, Normal School students, nurses, Indians and half-breeds; studies of infection and disease in different age groups; causes of tuberculosis among young adult women and men; and effectiveness of BCG vaccine).
- Adequate sanatorium beds (the only setback was the lack of a convalescent building).

The final plan for increased detection of undiagnosed tuberculosis concentrated on patients admitted to general hospitals, "since the incidence of tuberculosis is much higher among the sick than among the well." Dr. John Orr obtained funds from the Saskatchewan Department of Public Health to purchase stationary photofluorographic units to obtain miniature chest films of each patient on admission to hospital. The first unit was installed in the Yorkton General Hospital in 1947. Smaller hospitals took full-size films with regular x-ray equipment.

Dr. Orr, after little more than three months as director of medical services, made mention in his first annual report of a promising new drug, streptomycin, which reduced the risk of surgery in the tuberculous patient and was effective in treating certain patients. The Ferguson era was over. He had met the challenges of drought, depression and war. The chemotherapy era was about to be ushered in.

Retirement

On the day of his retirement, his sixty-fifth birthday, 12 September 1948, six hundred former patients gathered to bid him farewell. The ceremonies were opened by His Honour the Lieutenant Governor of Saskatchewan Dr. J.M. Uhrich, in earlier years the sympathetic minister of health. There was a welcome from Dr. John Orr, an address by League President E.G. Hingley, and remarks by Dr. G.J. Wherrett of Ottawa, executive director of the Canadian Tuberculosis Association. Mrs. Ken More made a presentation to Mrs. Ferguson. E.C. Leslie, K.C., gave Ferguson a purse of $2,500 from the League. The main address was given by the Hon. T.C. Douglas, premier of Saskatchewan and minister of health. John Fisher, the noted Canadian Broadcasting Corporation commentator, broadcast over the national radio network from the sanatorium grounds his regular twelve-minute coast-to-coast program "John Fisher Reports." The broadcast was devoted entirely to the life and work of Dr. Ferguson.

Ferguson's contemporaries, Kirkby, Boughton and Orr, all continued to work beyond retirement age. Apart from increasing frustrations, Ferguson had another good reason for retiring at age sixty-five: he wished to write the story of his life's crusade against tuberculosis.

Studies in Tuberculosis

In six retirement years, Ferguson wrote *Studies in Tuberculosis*. During the first winter, he spent several months at library research in Toronto, with a secretary provided by the Canadian Tuberculosis Association. In spite of his age and declining energy, he persevered. The book was published by the University of Toronto Press in 1955, aided by a subsidy from the Canadian Tuberculosis Association.

The 124-page book, which sold for $3.50, was divided into sixteen chapters, covering the ebb and flow of epidemics, non-specific resistance, racial susceptibility, family susceptibility, physiological factors, age and mortality, effect of population movement on a tuberculosis epidemic, elimination of susceptibles in attainment of resistance, bovine tuberculosis, severity of infection, sensitivity to tuberculo-protein, resistance, the course of tuberculosis epidemics, prevention of human tuberculosis, and rehabilitation. There were five pages of appendices and four of references.

In the foreword, Dr. N.E. McKinnon said that readers "will find in it more than a series of studies in tuberculosis. They will find in it the reflection of a way of life, a disregard for complacency, and a constant struggle for the truth."

Studies in Tuberculosis received favourable reviews. Both *Tubercle*, published in Great Britain, and the *American Journal of Public Health* were complimentary. The reviewer in the latter journal wrote:

> This book should be required reading for every student in public health, including public health nurses . . . This extremely intimate lifelong study with its thoroughness gives the necessary basic knowledge in which one can understand the role of mass studies and statistics in such a medical program . . . the author has understood the total problem of tuberculosis . . . one cannot read this book without getting a deeper insight into the seemingly endless battle against the disease.

The statement from the publishers, eighteen months after printing, showed that 510 copies had been produced at a cost of $1,475.98, $1,000 of this being covered by the subsidy, and the 367 copies sold at an average wholesale return of $2.78 had yielded revenue of $1,021.56. The Press took a 30 percent commission, and sent a royalty cheque of $239.11 to the author, who characteristically turned it over to the League.

While in active practice, Ferguson received many honours, which included presidency of the Saskatchewan Medical Association, member of the Senate of the University of Saskatchewan, Chief Muskeke-O-Kemacan (Great White Physician) by the Qu'Appelle Valley Indians, Order of the British Empire, and LL.D. (Honorary) from the University of Saskatchewan.[1] He was also elected an honorary life member of the Royal Canadian Legion in recognition of the great assistance he gave the tuberculous veterans of two world wars. On 25 April 1948 the Sacred Heart Scholasticate at Lebret gave an organ recital for two hundred guests in honour of Dr. and Mrs. Ferguson, at which Father Julien Morin, a former patient, read the address of appreciation.

Ferguson's most prestigious award was the Charles Mickle Fellowship in 1961, which carried a cash award of $1,200. The fellowship, established in 1921 by a bequest from Dr. William Julius Mickle, is awarded to the person who in the opinion of the Faculty of Medicine, University of Toronto, has done most during the preceding ten years to advance sound knowledge of a practical kind in medical art or science. A list of winners before Ferguson is a veritable who's who in medicine, and contains, among other renowned names, Ivan Petrovich Pavlov of conditioned reflex fame, Harvey Williams Cushing, Boston neurosurgeon, and (Sir) Frederick Grant Banting, co-discoverer of insulin. In 1962, a group from Regina commissioned his portrait by Nicholas de Grandmaison, an artist from Banff, Alberta, who shared Ferguson's love and respect for Plains Indians. His name is perpetuated in the Dr. George Ferguson Public School at 117 Brotherton Avenue, Regina, and in a large island in Montreal Lake, Saskatchewan.

R.G. Ferguson Professorship, University of Saskatchewan

The Wherrett-Grzybowski report of 1966 recommended close integration between the College of Medicine and the Saskatoon Sanatorium. Negotiations between Dr. G.D. Barnett and Frank Froh of the League and Drs. A.A. Bailey and L. Horlick of the university began in 1969, but the appointment to the newly established R.G. Ferguson professorship was delayed until 1972, when a suitable chest physician was recruited and a clinical research laboratory in respiratory diseases established. The League agreed to contribute financially towards the development of the research laboratory and to the professorship, and has continued to give about a quarter of a million dollars each year to the special chest disease unit at the Royal University Hospital. Dr. Jim Dosman held the R.G. Ferguson professorship from 1972 and was followed by Dr. David Cotton in 1984 and by Dr. Vern Hoeppner in 1986. The direction, quality and quantity of research in the unit is a worthy memorial to Ferguson and his work.

After *Studies in Tuberculosis* was published, Ferguson showed increasing signs of age. He and Mrs. Ferguson continued to spend their summers at their cottage at Echo Lake near the sanatorium and their winters in the Balfour Apartments in Regina, where she hid as best she could his decreasing mental powers.

After a short illness Ferguson died at the age of eighty in the Regina General Hospital, 1 March 1964. Over seven hundred people crowded Knox Metropolitan Church in Regina for the funeral on 4 March. Among those who attended to pay their last respects were Lieutenant Governor R.L. Hanbidge; former premier and former lieutenant governor W.J. Patterson; former premier and former chief justice W.M. Martin; Health Minister Allan Blakeney; and Regina's member of Parliament, Ken More. Ferguson was buried at Fort Qu'Appelle. "His resting place is in the valley he loved, but his shrine is in the hearts of the people of Saskatchewan."[2]

— Chapter Eight —

Man With a Mission

WHEN HE WAS thirteen, George attended a Methodist revival meeting in South Joliette School. The evangelist's message was that individuals must learn to control their tempers. Those with undisciplined tempers were called to move forward in public confession and prayer. The desperately shy George realized that, like his father, he had an unbridled temper; he found the courage to step forward to repent. Henceforward he had the strength to master his temper "except when he encountered injustice."

George attended Salvation Army services in the old South Joliette school, led by Lieutenant Hector Habkirk, brother of the Salvationist who wrote the Army song, "We'll Roll The Old Chariots Along." Though Ferguson in the end abandoned his plans for the Methodist ministry, he remained throughout his life a man with a mission.

When they speak about their father now, his children recall the combination of love and religious faith that was his strength. His daughter Sheelagh Ferguson Barrable remembers the touching present she received from her father at Christmas when she was twelve – a pastel sketch made by her mother of herself and her twin brother, from a photograph taken just before he died. On the back of the picture was written a simple, homespun poem, composed by her father in November 1926 to console his wife in her grief. It ended with two lines of unflagging faith:

> Life's stern separations and unfulfilled plans
> Are perfection to God who alone understands.

Sheelagh recalls, "The tears flowed down my cheeks as I sensed the faith with which that poem had been written. It remains to this day my most cherished gift, for it was truly a gift of abiding faith in the presence of God."

As a Methodist student minister, Ferguson preached of a God whose presence could be felt by anyone who had faith; faith had to be nurtured for it to grow and develop. On Sunday he held prayers in his home, with everyone kneeling. He had a life-long desire to re-write the Lord's Prayer to include "to forgive is to forget," a presumption which would have seemed pretentious had it not so movingly revealed his innocence and the depth of his sincerity.

Ferguson's life was a fulfilment of the two great Christian commandments, to love God and to love your fellow man. In the early years at the San, he faced death with each dying patient, sharing his faith and courage with them. Bible reading and prayer were part of his life, but as he became busier he did not attend the weekly church service as regularly, for example, as Dr. Boughton. Ferguson felt personal experience was more important than institutionalized religion, and believed everyone should formulate his own relationship with God. Testimonials to his beliefs were written in private confessions to his family

My God

As God was revealed to me from infancy by life and Christ, I built unto myself a God of many attributes.

A God of home – a mother-father God

- I run home to be cuddled
- I run home to rest
- I run home to eat – a providing God (seasons, rain, harvest)

A God of protection – a big brother God

- shows us how to handle big problems
- protects us against enemies and adversaries
- pulls us out of difficulties

A God of character and worth

- wise, understanding, honest and just
- a respected creator and co-ordinator
- a source of peace
- a source of power
- the spirit pervading the universe
- a source of the spirit breathed into man as the breath of life and limited divinity

A God of adoration

- the God I love – per Augustine of Hippo:
  "the sum total of what I can conceive as the highest in quality and worth. Not grace of body or harmony of time, nor gladness, nor sweet melodies of song, nor fragrance of flowers, nor manna or honey; yet I love a kind of light melody, fragrance, food of the inner man, where there shinest into my soul what space cannot contain and there soundest what time beareth not away. This is what I love when I love my God."

Ferguson's Philosophy

At Creation, God breathed into man the breath of life, "The Spirit." At the first quickening of the womb there is breathed into the creature the breath, the limited spirit of the Deity.

At death, there departs from the creature, the breath, the limited spirit of the Deity. This finite spirit, now in reverse, with its love of God, its sense of worth, its desire for protection, its homing instinct, returns to the Creator, to God. "Where I am, there ye may be also" (John 14:3).

There is a strong desire of many men both ancient and modern, to live after death. This may be due to the homing instinct of the finite spirit of man. Heaven is the return to God, the reversion of the finite spirit to the infinite spirit. The location of Heaven is everywhere and anywhere. I am happy in him.

God is good. Life is sweet. Struggling, toiling, rejoicing and sorrowing develops character. Contemplation and prayer develops the appreciation for quality and value. Adoration, love of God, develops the finite spirit of God in man. Following Christ develops man in the image of God.

Although man is spiritually endowed with the infinite spirit of God, still he is biologically a selfish survivalist. The selfless and altruistic strains have frequently been eliminated in the struggle to survive.

As civilization improves, more selfless and altruistic strains survive and progress is slowly made toward sociological improvement of the race. On the contrary, it may be that artificial efforts to increase resistance against disease and lessen the struggle may lead to the survival of inferior strains, thus weakening the biological character of the race.

The period of physical and intellectual development of man is brief and the life cycle is short; nevertheless the efficiency of development and education can be increased so as to raise the average in the limited time available. This is a passive improvement, confined to its generalities, that would subside with reduced effort.

The kinship of spiritually finite man and spiritually infinite God is fundamental and indestructible; where material needs are reasonably attained and qualities and values are appreciated, at this point man will seek higher spiritual attainments.

Ferguson's Creed

God is my Father.
I will endeavour to honour His commandments.
Jesus is my Saviour and my guide.
I will strive with His help
To follow His example and His teachings,
To pray as He taught me to pray,
To forgive others as He has forgiven me,
To commemorate His presence and eternal
sacrifice by the Sacrament of the Lord's Supper.

To Ferguson and his contemporaries there would have been nothing trite or sanctimonious in R.W. Kirkby's exhortation when he opened the Prince Albert Sanatorium:

Do all the good you can,
To all the people you can,
In all the ways you can,
As long as ever you can.

George and Helen Ferguson were devoted to each other and their "chubbs." Their home was a warm and loving place where friends of their children were always welcome; George was never too busy to have a "wee chat" with each visitor. Only when Helen wasn't home would he visit the neighbours – a sure sign of her absence.

Ferguson would hug his sons and daughters regardless of their age, to the embarrassment of at least one visitor, David B. Stewart, when he was a young lad. Ferguson children were a captive audience in the breakfast nook, from which their only escape was by climbing behind one another. Here he would tell them stories about Euripides, Ulysses, Penelope, and of Pheidippides who ran the twenty-six miles from Marathon to Athens. He wanted each to develop his or her own philosophy of life as a guide for the rough spots ahead.

As Ferguson told his children, a painful experience could be turned to their benefit. He had experienced much sorrow himself. Before leaving North Dakota he had lost two brothers, one in an accident and one from diphtheria, and a sister had died from tuberculosis. Another brother had been killed in World War I, and a second, who had been gassed in the war, died from tuberculosis. His father had died before his new farm was well established, and his mother had become blind.

Her father had beautiful gifts to offer, Patricia says. "A kindly, gentle humour; a deep gratitude for his blessings; a keen sense of the importance of good attitudes; a deep understanding of human frailties; forgiveness and forgetness; joy of learning; fortitude of perseverance and stamina; courage in the face of the impossible."

William Houston, of the investment firm Houston & Willoughby, came to visit Ferguson soon after his wife Elsie had died following a lingering illness. Patricia remembers the day, Ferguson and Houston sitting side-by-side, the physician and his bereaved friend. For a long time, neither said a word. Patricia was witnessing the meaning of true friendship, as she had never understood it before. There was no need for words – only the silence of shared grief in mutual mourning.

Ferguson quickly grasped complicated issues and explained them in simple terms. He treated problems with cool sanity, quiet discussion and an attentive ear. He could get along with the most difficult people and see the good side of each. He never gossiped and never judged aloud. High spirits could make him almost kittenish, as when he did a little dance in the kitchen before setting off with the family on a one-day holiday. But normally his was a quiet sense of humour, as when he told his children to remember his example when they came to choose a spouse. He had looked for a people-person with a lot of character, a woman who would be diplomatic, a good hostess, hospitable, loving, kind, generous, loyal – yet, said he, beauty was not a qualification: he could supply that!

Patricia saw tears run down her father's cheeks only three times. The first, when he told her about the 1890 depression and the death of his brother and sister, Herby Wesley and Ida May. Then there was Father Athol Murray's struggles to keep Notre Dame College at Wilcox alive during the Depression. The last was when he was ill in bed and Patricia entered the sick room, to hear her father read aloud the last pages of Lloyd C. Douglas's *The Robe*.

Ferguson read widely in politics and economics, yet remained scrupulously non-political. His family and friends never knew which political party he supported. He enjoyed *Candide* and humourous stories by Damon Runyon in *Wilbur Is Wonderful*, also Schulberg's *What Makes Sammy Run*. When he was reading his power of concentration was absolute. A call to the dinner table rarely registered, so one of the children would go over to his easy chair and tap him on the shoulder to get his attention.

He was a teetotaller and allowed no liquor in the home. A boyfriend of one of his daughters once brought a bottle of liquor to the house at Christmas; it was poured down the drain.

He admonished his children: "Stay out of debt; to owe money is akin to stealing; education offers lifetime protection; work hard, never stop trying; never lose faith in people or carry a grudge; selfishness is man's greatest sin; the happiest and most fulfilling occupations are those that offer service to others."

He would ask, "What kind thing have you done today?"

Ferguson's compassion was central to his character. During the Depression a man arrived by train and made his way out to Ferguson's office at Fort San where he tried to sell Ferguson some shares in a brewery. Ferguson quietly told the salesman that he never purchased liquor or stocks. Noting that the salesman looked pale and tired, he took him to the Red Cross Lodge and arranged for his supper, a night's lodging, and breakfast. The next morning he drove him to the CNR station to catch the train back to Regina. At supper Ferguson lectured his children, "Never make your living from the production or sale of liquor. People in such an occupation are partly responsible for the break-up of homes, battering of wives and children, deep insecurity of growing children, and divorce." A week later, the man was found dead in a hotel room in Weyburn.

The Fergusons provided a home for Helen's parents, Mr. and Mrs. Hervey Ross, for years. Grandfather Hervey Ross died on 8 March 1928.

Although he was an insurance salesman, he had no life insurance himself. Grandmother Ross lived with the Fergusons year-round until she died on 26 March 1934.

Ferguson also contributed to the support of his mother, who outlived his father by more than forty years. Undeterred by painful glaucoma, which eventually made her blind, she took a typing course so she could continue to correspond with her friends. Friends and family read to her and after their visits she would speak of having "seen" them. When she moved off the farm she rented a house at 43 Agricultural Avenue, in Yorkton, from J.A.M. Patrick. In 1935 she joined her daughter, Laura Ruttle, on a farm at Fone Hill, ten miles west of Yorkton, until her death on 21 January 1948. She was survived by three sons, six daughters, thirty-five grandchildren, twenty-eight great-grandchildren and two great-great-grandchildren.

George and Helen Ferguson's children never heard their mother raise her voice, or say anything unkind about anyone, or indulge in gossip. When children were ill, she was a natural nurse, with a knack for making them feel better, since she had the "kindest hands" Patricia ever knew. Dick Motherwell, Patricia's husband, said his mother-in-law was the kindest woman he had ever met.

A gracious hostess, Helen did a great deal of formal and informal entertaining. There was always a welcome mat at the door, even for those who arrived unannounced. George, who was shy, depended on her for the ice-breaking at social gatherings.

A regular part of the Ferguson Christmas was the arrival of the Indian chief, Towweeaka, from the Sioux reserve six miles away. He was always invited in to see the tree, sit awhile, share a smoke with Dr. Ferguson, and meet the guests. He left with a bag of gifts to take back to the reserve. The year that Towweeaka was too ill to come, three runners arrived in his place and received the usual gifts. After Christmas, Ferguson went out to the reserve to visit the old chief before he died.

Helen Ferguson loved to be surrounded by beauty. She was a talented artist who took painting lessons from James Henderson, RCA. Her favourite subjects were valley scenes and portraits; she even painted a portrait of James Henderson. When she was in Toronto while George was doing research there in the winter after his retirement, she studied painting under Cleeve Horne. After a short course in sculpting in Saskatoon, she executed a remarkable life-size bust of her husband

and six smaller busts, one for each child. She designed the Ferguson cedar-log cabin, just over a mile from the sanatorium on Echo Lake, and graced the great stone fireplace with her cedar carving of an Indian head.

Helen worked hard looking after her large family and huge garden. Dancing, singing and sewing were among her favourite pastimes. She made costumes for the Hallowe'en Evening in the San auditorium. She was not an avid reader and did not care for solitary activities. She preferred horse-riding, canoeing, golf, curling, skating, tobogganing, bobsledding, tennis and ping-pong. She even shot ducks and pheasants.

When holidays came round all six children were packed into the car – Mother, Dad and Robert in the front seat, Helen, Margaret and Patricia in the back, with David and Sheelagh precariously perched on the front of the back seat between them. Tent and bedding were stowed on top of the car, food and utensils on the right-hand running-board and clothes in the trunk. They made their own meals as they travelled on their week-long trips to Waskesiu, Banff, Waterton, Cypress Hills, and Vancouver.

Sheelagh wrote to her eighty-nine-year-old mother on Thanksgiving Day, 1981, recalling earlier times:

> Just looking out of my bedroom window I can see the golden bronze of the maple trees and it makes me think of you. A little squirrel just went scampering by and he makes me think of how busy you were for most of your wonderful life. The babies that you fed and loved, the bottoms that you spanked and the tears that you kissed away . . . You moulded and loved and forgave and nurtured all your life . . . How very blessed were we six chubbies to be born to one who loved us so completely that she could forgive us all our faults . . . The amazing thing about it was that you still had time to express your creative talents, both in oils and sculpturing. You have added so much joy and pleasure to our lives by your interest in all that was beautiful. Each one of us has treasures that you have skillfully created. Everywhere I look in my home there is a little bit of you . . . Our security was based on the fact that we knew without a shadow of a doubt that our parents not only loved us but that they loved one another with a strength that made us all feel

> secure . . . you kept the atmosphere in our home a happy positive one that we loved to come home to . . . your energy was prodigious; there isn't one of us in the family who could keep up to the pace that you set. I remember the summer I spent at home before I joined the service and you wore me out by four in the afternoon and when I was ready to collapse you would suggest nine holes of golf. Truly darling you lived life to the full . . . May God bless and keep you safe always.

Ferguson's personality and varied skills were as impressive as his medical achievements. His accomplishments would have been considered remarkable even in a more affluent province where private wealth was available to be tapped. They were particularly impressive in an agrarian society hampered by a perennial shortage of funds. Ferguson's success was in large part due to his personal approach, his methods, and his resourcefulness.

Tuberculosis was the greatest public health problem of the time and the second commonest cause of death, yet the predominant attitude towards it was defeatist. Almost every member of society became infected with tuberculosis at some time during life, and many would succumb. Most doctors had a fatalistic approach towards the disease. In England, for example, the value of sanatoria was seriously questioned, especially after Sir George Newman in 1920 found three-quarters of the patients admitted to English sanatoria died within five years. Little could be done to prevent exposure and there was less to offer in the way of specific treatment. Most patients had infected others before their own tuberculosis had been diagnosed.

In spite of the near-hopeless outlook, Ferguson galvanized, educated, and cajoled an entire province. Nowhere else did the attack on tuberculosis, or perhaps any other single disease, have so much grassroots support. The necessary facilities were disproportionate in size and cost for a poor province; Saskatchewan was one of the least likely jurisdictions to have led North America.[1]

Ferguson organized a populist, cooperative, province-wide effort to raise money for the League and to keep public concern alive. Often the responses were simple but symbolic. Groups of farmer's wives, scattered throughout the province and organized as Homemakers' Clubs, would each donate dozens of eggs or chickens to feed the patients. Radio announcers gave their time to put on weekly amateur shows. Just about everyone got involved – schoolchildren, teachers, nurses, doctors, and key organizations in each community. For years there was an essay contest for school children. Prospective teachers were taught about tuberculosis at Normal Schools.

In a predominantly rural province, Ferguson understood farmers and spoke their language. He represented the anti-tuberculosis campaign by an agrarian metaphor in his 1942 annual report:

> The people of Saskatchewan know that tuberculosis is a bad weed. In the language of the farmer, it is a perennial which, if not uprooted, will shed its seeds from year to year. When these weeds or cases are sparse the best practice is to find them and remove them before the seeds are shed. To do this everyone must learn to identify tuberculosis in the seed, in the sprout, in the leaf, in the flower, or in the ripe shelling. That is why the educational campaign for the prevention of tuberculosis goes on in schools, Normal Schools, families, communities, and throughout the province generally. From past results our people have the faith, confidence and will to eradicate this disease. Come peace, come war, prosperity or depression, this life-saving campaign goes on, resulting in less infection, less new cases, and in the end less deaths.

Ferguson had the full support of the League's dedicated Board of Directors. Peter McAra continued on the Board of Directors after he stepped down as first president, and he served again as president from 1930 to 1941. E.G. Hingley represented the Saskatchewan Association of Rural Municipalities for forty years and was president of the League from 1945 until his death in 1958. Dr. F.W. Hart of Indian Head, an original trustee from 1911 to 1918, returned to the board as representative of the Saskatchewan Medical Association from 1932 to 1946. His son, Bob, married Ferguson's daughter, Helen.

Ferguson's timing, too, was perfect. World War I had changed public attitudes more than anyone realized; few other "charities" had so much appeal. As his mentor, Dr. David A. Stewart, so forcibly argued before the Anti-tuberculosis Society in Winnipeg:

> The war had led us to the verge of a new conception regarding illness, its care and cure. If the wounded or tuberculous soldier

> be cared for until he is well, or helped indefinitely if he should not return to complete health, it is not difficult to argue that the soldier of commerce, or industry, or of agriculture, when disabled, should be cared for in the same way. If the man who fights abroad is to be provided for in illness, why not the woman whose work and child-bearing have broken her down at home; and why not the child, the worker?

All three sanatoria took great care to maintain good relationships with practising doctors. As Boughton said later, "One of his long suits was to play hand-in-glove with the doctors who referred patients . . . Should there have been delay in suspecting tuberculosis he would find an explanation so that the family would maintain confidence in its doctor." In other parts of Canada, Ferguson was sometimes the butt for his failure to enlist a field nursing staff, but he countered, "We can't go over the heads of family doctors. What we need is patients, and who will find them but the doctors? So we'll play ball with the family doctors." This was one of the reasons why Saskatchewan was quick off the mark in its highly successful campaign against tuberculosis.

In the early years Ferguson made sure that both legislators and doctors were familiar with the sanatorium and its work. On 26 November 1920 he gave a tour of the sanatorium to thirty members of the Legislative Assembly, and in June 1922 the Saskatchewan Medical Association held its annual meeting at the Fort Qu'Appelle Sanatorium.

Whether the Liberals or Conservatives were in power, Ferguson had immediate access to the premier and the minister of public health. He consistently gained maximum government support. Yet he kept a tight rein on management. There was no patronage and no featherbedding. The League gave in service to the public a great deal more for each dollar than if the sanatoria had been run by the government bureaucracy. The League, followed by the Saskatchewan Lung Association, was allowed to operate the sanatoria and clinics, the entire tuberculosis program, until 1987. Members of each successive government realized, sometimes contrary to dogma, that the arrangement was mutually beneficial. The various levels of government put up the money while the League ran the show, with a great deal of help from many volunteers and private organizations. At the same time the League attracted exceptionally dedicated people and provided a high standard of care.

The sanatorium staff did not benefit from the pension plans available to those directly employed by government. In the early years the young, idealistic and enthusiastic staff gave little thought to pensions until the need became apparent at the very depth of the Depression. Yet Ferguson, in spite of the difficult times, managed to have a sanatorium superannuation bill passed by the legislature early in 1935, to come into force on 1 March 1935. By modern standards, the pensions were not generous, consisting of 2 percent of final salary multiplied by years of service. The minimum annual pension was $360 and the maximum was $2,000. At the time, $4,000 would purchase a nice home. In retirement, Ferguson received $166.66 per month from his League pension; after his death, his widow received $83.33 per month, later increased to $166.66 from League funds.

Ferguson earned the respect of all major politicians of his time. But he also had the good fortune to have personal friends within the provincial cabinet and the House of Commons.

It was a happy accident that the sanatorium was strategically situated within provincial and federal constituencies usually represented by influential politicians. Federally, the riding of Melville was represented by W.R. Motherwell, an Abernethy farmer, from 1925 to 1940. For ten years before Motherwell's marriage, his wife, Kate Gillespie, had been principal of the school on the File Hills Indian Reserve. She had a powerful faith in the Indians, and her husband and Ferguson often sought her advice. Motherwell had been an influential provincial cabinet minister who had met with the League executive on the first day of its existence in 1911. He was Saskatchewan's minister of agriculture when the first attempts to control bovine tuberculosis were made, offering free tuberculin testing and creating "T.B. restricted areas." Later, as Liberal minister of agriculture in the House of Commons, Motherwell used his influence to get his friend, Dr. Austin Simes of nearby Abernethy, Saskatchewan, appointed as Indian health doctor, so that Simes and Ferguson could do important research together. Motherwell, though on the opposition side of the House, had some influence in persuading the government to build a new Indian hospital in Fort Qu'Appelle in 1936, mainly for the treatment of tuberculosis. The relationship was further strengthened when Ferguson's daughter Patricia married the Motherwells' grandson.

Provincially, the sanatorium was within the constituency of North Qu'Appelle, represented by James G. Gardiner from 1914 to 1934, and, after redistribution, within the newly formed Melville constituency, also represented by Gardiner in 1934–35. Ferguson and Gardiner had been classmates at Wesley College in Winnipeg. Gardiner was premier of Saskatchewan from 1926 to 1929 and again in 1934–35, before he switched to federal politics to become federal minister of agriculture. He had won Assiniboia in a by-election, but returned to represent the federal constituency of Melville, which included the sanatorium, from 1940 to 1958. The presence of the sanatorium within the riding of a provincial premier who later became a major federal cabinet minister, together with the fact that Gardiner's first wife had died of tuberculosis, assured Ferguson of sympathetic support from the provincial and federal governments.

Ferguson was also fortunate in that T.C. Douglas kept the important health portfolio himself when he became the first CCF premier of the province. Douglas, having spent much of his youth in hospital with chronic osteomyelitis, was particularly sympathetic to health needs. Ferguson's projects were no flash-in-the-pan enthusiasms; they lasted through drought, depression and war in spite of competition from other worthy causes. Money was raised in increasing amounts as it was needed.

Until 1945 no federal financial assistance had been available to the sanatoria, apart from a major commitment to care for tuberculous servicemen after each war. When Saskatchewan became eligible for a tuberculosis grant that year, its share was $180,000 from $3 million in national funds.

In all three sanatoria the doctors, nurses and orderlies provided a consistently high standard of loving care, unusual for such large institutions. Ferguson, his doctors and nurses set the tone and all employees lived up to this example. As with most doctors of the era, devotion and dedication were taken for granted, while monetary considerations were secondary.

Of the many selfless staff members attracted by Ferguson, orderly Alf Johnson deserves special mention. With his personal motto, "Nothing is too good for the patients," and out of his meagre income, he bought paper and stamps, chocolate bars and radios and at Christmas cooked a turkey or a goose for patients whose morale needed a boost. Throughout each day he encouraged and joked with patients, then returned after duty to make tea and toast. He performed his inimitable

English music hall routines at every concert. During the war he served as orderly with the Winnipeg Grenadiers, spending nearly four years of misery in Japanese prisoner-of-war camps, but returned to complete thirty-six years of service at Fort San.

Long-term incarceration of patients was in many ways worse than prison, especially for North American Indians. Much thought and ingenuity went into the effort to make each patient happy, contented and part of the family, during long periods in hospital, which sometimes stretched to five years or more. At the same time, discipline was strict. If a patient with "open" tuberculosis escaped (or "eloped," to use the quaint euphemism of the day), the Royal Canadian Mounted Police were notified that the patient was a risk to society. The patient was brought back, much as if he had escaped from prison.

Veronica Eddy Brock's semi-autobiographical story, *Valley of the Flowers*, published in 1986, shocked many of Ferguson's admirers. Life in the San, as portrayed by Brock, was not a bed of roses. In her teens, skinny but in apparent good health, she was plucked out of high school and incarcerated for years in a sanatorium, where one lung was removed. Yet she did not harbour a grudge against her doctors, as many readers had inferred by reading between the lines. Not at all. Dr. Louis Wettlaufer was her doctor and she couldn't imagine having anyone finer. She recalled that Dr. Ferguson, though in charge of tuberculosis for the entire province, made rounds to visit every patient each Sunday, escorted by Mrs. Ferguson, whose social skills made it possible for her to know every patient by name.

It was a matter of pride each year that Saskatchewan consistently recorded a lower tuberculosis death rate than any other province. Not until 1941 did Ontario take the lead, only to lose it to Saskatchewan for one last time in 1942.

No matter what burdens he carried, Ferguson took his time, patiently, with the person or the matter at hand. Hard times, war, adversity of any kind, failed to deter him. New programs went ahead during wartime in spite of a shortage of staff and materials. He harnessed the services of a great many volunteers in each community to ensure continuance of the radiographic surveys.

As Professor Dorothy Kline, once a patient with spinal tuberculosis, has said, "His dogged determination in the face of almost insurmountable difficulties and his ability to accept the inevitable while focusing his energy on improvement of the attainable, were at once inspiration and strength to those about him."[2]

In Dr. G.J. Wherrett's words:

> His natural inclination to excuse the failings of others made some of us wonder if at times he put a premium on mediocrity and inefficiency. Later we were to realize that this was the secret of his success . . . he obtained each person's best efforts, irrespective of his ability. The loyalty to his staff aroused the kindred loyalty to himself which was shown by all who worked with him. His ability to appreciate another's point of view added to the power of persuasion for which he was noted . . . He was not an eloquent speaker, and in the main stuck closely to his text, but his sincerity and sensitivity were so striking that his words made a vivid and lasting impression.

As Boughton remarked:

> In matters of institutional discipline he was always putting himself in the other fellow's shoes, rarely making hasty decisions, but always commanding respect . . . Often to the chagrin of members of his staff he would spend unconscionable time closeted with someone who was not considered worthy of so much attention.
>
> If he sensed that certain members of the Board of Directors "might not see eye to eye with him," he would find occasion to casually meet them, lay out his plan, discuss it and leave the matter without trying to obtain their approval. Time was always on his side . . . Eventually . . . the dissident members, finding they knew more of the matter than most of the Board, would become "yes" men. Surely this was a master manoeuvre resulting in having nearly all the Board members supporting him nearly all the time; and certainly no one ever heard a Board member publicly opposing him.

As Kirkby observed:

> He possessed the faculty of getting people to go along with him in a greater degree than anyone I have ever known, he had that

> certain something which most executives lack, a clear understanding of the relation between cause and effect. He explained what he had in mind and sold his point of view to you. His ability to enlist the whole-hearted effort of those around him was to me the keynote of his success.

Ferguson was unusual in according research such a high priority. The output of first-class scientific papers emanating from the sanatorium was creditable for an institution in a rural setting, far from a university and several days' train travel from major centres, at a time when long-distance telephone calls were made sparingly. Fort San accumulated the best medical library in Saskatchewan to facilitate his research. Surprisingly, in spite of his literary output, he was an abysmal speller.

Ferguson's output of scientific papers, an extensive commission report and a book, was an exceptional achievement for a man heavily committed to patient care and administrative duties. The use he made of statistical methodology was unusual in the 1930s. He encouraged and cajoled staff members into completing research studies which supplemented his own. Several papers, notably those by Iva Molony in 1928 and W.S. Barclay in 1931, won the $250 annual prize of the Canadian Tuberculosis Association for the best paper by a staff member with less than five years' experience. Charles F. Bennett's paper in 1935 also won a CTA prize.

The scientific community was not the only beneficiary of his knowledge. Ferguson wrote forty-four articles and twenty-two annual reports for the *Valley Echo*, explaining aspects of tuberculosis to patients and their families. Boughton, Kirkby, Hamilton, and Orr wrote many other articles for the monthly.

Ferguson was unusually successful in attracting and keeping staff of the highest quality. Late in his career he heard of Jim Romeyn, a Canadian studying in England, who had the special experience needed by the League. He made arrangements to interview him, though he had been warned Romeyn had once been a card-carrying Communist. "His politics don't matter," he said, "if he is a first-class medical doctor."

Ferguson's reputation was such that almost no one would think of opposing him on any matter. He acquired special privileges usually reserved for a state dignitary. The Canadian National Railways more than once held a train for him when his secretary phoned to say Dr. Ferguson had been delayed. Few policemen had the temerity to stop

Mrs. Ferguson for speeding, though she was notorious for exceeding the speed limit once the highway to Regina had been paved.

His faults were minor and excusable. His absentmindedness twice caused his suspension (later forgiven) from the Rotary Club in Fort Qu'Appelle for not attending their Monday evening meetings. Sometimes he was out of town, sometimes he didn't care to go, but often he simply forgot what evening it was. Stories, which may or may not be apocryphal, include the one about his driving back from Regina without his wife because he had forgotten she had gone with him. Once he took the League's blue car to the legislative grounds, driving home in another which, by chance, accepted the same ignition key. The episode appeared in the *Regina Leader-Post* under the headline DOCTOR STEALS CAR.

He did not take to social niceties easily. His mother had not succeeded in teaching him that boys hold the door open for girls, and that a man should help a woman into a chair. Guests in his home were embarrassed when the visiting husband held the chair at the table for Mrs. Ferguson while the visiting wife received no such courtesy. He never remembered a birthday or anniversary. He was not athletic, and could always think of a good reason not to curl, golf, swim, or play tennis. He went hunting in his early years, but was a poor shot. He had a reputation for always bidding "three no trump" when he played bridge. He relates in a letter to his children how such a bid occasionally paid off: "The other evening we found ourselves in the company of carefree gamblers, where to get in on the game I was forced to over-bid and fortune favored me to the extent of three successful finesses, entitling me to the fruits of a vulnerable three no trump, doubled, so you see I am still playing with small cards."

— Chapter Nine —

Postscript

AFTER HIS RETIREMENT Ferguson watched with amazement and pleasure the sudden and drastic improvement in the treatment of tuberculosis; streptomycin, PAS (para-aminosalicyclic acid), INH (isonicotinic acid hydrazide) and other new anti-tuberculosis drugs appeared in turn. Instead of slow, faltering progress, effective treatment advanced rapidly. Surgery, also more successful, was needed less often. The death rate dropped quickly.

Streptomycin had been isolated in January 1944 by Selman A. Waksman. Sufficient quantities of this difficult-to-prepare and expensive drug became available for use in Saskatchewan sanatoria on 1 April 1948. The second drug, PAS, was added later that year. Beginning on 15 July 1948, free distribution of streptomycin to sanatoria through federal health grants quickly resulted in its widespread use.

During the year before streptomycin was distributed, Saskatchewan's death rate had dropped as much in a single year as in the ten previous years – from 26.1 to 21.5 per 100,000. Aided by the use of streptomycin in selected patients, the death rate the following year dropped to 18.5 (11 per 100,000 for the white population alone). Community surveys were accelerated so that the second round, photofluorography of 640,348 individuals, was completed by June 1950. Nevertheless, there were still 415 new active cases of tuberculosis and 153 deaths in Saskatchewan in 1950.

The yield from community photofluorographic surveys fell rapidly. In 1951, from 238,000 miniature radiographs, only sixty-seven new cases of tuberculosis were discovered, barely half the number found two years earlier. A greater yield was available from the hospital admission radiographs, with ninety-one new cases discovered in 1952, one for each 727 films taken. Over one-third of the positive radiographs were from two of the smaller hospitals that served native populations, La Loche and Île-à-la-Crosse. The bad news was that Saskatchewan's Indian tuberculosis death rate was still 273.5 per 100,000 population in 1952, worse than Canada's average Indian death rate, 167.5, for that year. Between 1949 and 1950, treatment days for Saskatchewan Indians jumped from 25,647 to 38,443. By the end of 1952, 194 Indians were under treatment in the three sanatoria, and thirty-seven in the Indian hospitals in Fort Qu'Appelle and North Battleford.

The sharp drop in the death rate was a worldwide phenomenon. Canada's death rate fell to a record low of 17.1 per 100,000 in 1952. Even better were Cyprus (8.0), Denmark (11.3), the Netherlands (12.3) and the United States (16.1). Saskatchewan's tuberculosis death rate was down to 4.8 in 1954, with only twelve Indians and thirty whites dying of the disease. By 1961 Canada's tuberculosis death rate was down to 4.2, though Saskatchewan, with three Indian and twenty-two white deaths, had slipped to third place among the ten provinces.

Canadian sanatoria reached their peak occupancy of 17,364 beds in 1953. By June 1955, there were 716 patients and sixty empty beds in the three Saskatchewan sanatoria. At the end of 1961, with the aid of streptomycin and after the Prince Albert Sanatorium had closed its doors, there were only 120 patients at Saskatoon and 96 at Fort San – although 146 new active cases had been discovered that year and another 75 former patients had required readmission. The fifth round of photofluorographic surveys was completed in 1962, by which date 79 percent of the population had been examined. Not one new active case of tuberculosis was discovered among the Indians at Beauval, Île-à-la-Crosse, Buffalo Narrows, Uranium City and Cumberland House, where 3,462 individuals had been radiographed. In 1963, only 4.4 percent of Saskatchewan children at the age of fourteen had a positive tuberculin test, though this was still four times higher than the idealistic World Health Organization goal of 1 percent for this age.

At the time of Ferguson's death in 1964 everyone was optimistic that the final eradication of tuberculosis was at hand, though Canada's native people, Indians and Inuit, were still afflicted by the disease at Third World levels.

In retrospect the optimism of 1964 was not warranted. Tuberculosis was still killing more North Americans than all other infectious diseases combined – 10,000 people yearly in the United States. Since then, drug resistance, lack of public appreciation of the need for continued vigilance, and apathy have combined to forestall the hoped-for elimination of TB. Instead, tuberculosis has resisted eradication; in most countries the incidence is again on the rise, particularly among patients who are HIV-positive with the AIDS virus.

Provinces which provided the most sanatorium beds had the lowest TB death rates, but the policy may not have been cost-effective.

Certainly, sanatorium treatment benefited many individuals and contained the spread of the disease from open cases. But statisticians point out today that, throughout the Western world, tuberculosis incidence rates and death rates were already falling before the days of sanatoria and continued to decline at a fairly steady rate. Was the apparent success of sanatoria in lowering these rates merely a slight acceleration of what would have occurred without them? There were no statistically controlled studies anywhere in the world that randomized patients for sanatorium treatment against home treatment. Nor were there controlled studies to determine the benefits, if any, of pneumothorax and thoracoplasty. At any rate, sanatoria are no longer needed to segregate patients with active disease, because chemotherapy makes most patients non-infectious within days or weeks of the onset of treatment.

Sanatoria have been dismantled in most countries. In 1981, in recognition of the diminishing demands of tuberculosis, the Anti-tuberculosis League became the Saskatchewan Lung Association; more time and money are now devoted to lung cancer and pulmonary emphysema.

On 1 August 1987 the Saskatchewan Department of Health relieved the Lung Association of its seventy-six-year commitment for the care of patients with tuberculosis; patients came directly under government responsibility. A laboratory microbiologist in Regina has replaced the doctor in charge of the tuberculosis program, but has help from the pulmonary medicine department at Royal University Hospital, Saskatoon.

A mechanism to ensure that tuberculous patients take the necessary drugs no longer exists. Patient compliance is often lacking. In 1986, when 668 asymptomatic patients with positive tuberculin reactions in northern Saskatchewan were offered simple, easy-to-take INH treatment, 410 declined and only 258 accepted the preventive treatment. Of these, 4 percent had drug toxicity and stopped the INH. Only 3 percent of those at risk took an adequate dose of INH for the entire year. Compliance in taking treatment drugs is hardly any better in native patients with active disease; 61 percent of patients in northern Saskatchewan did not complete their treatment. Drugs then become ineffective because inadequate therapy allows surviving bacilli to develop drug resistance.

Recent tuberculosis statistics are discouraging. Saskatchewan in 1987 had 141 new patients with tuberculosis, sixteen relapses and five deaths. The incidence rates were ethnically disproportionate: 156 per 100,000 for Métis, 140 for Asians, 114 for native Indians and only 2.4 per 100,000 for Caucasians. Three native children had widespread tuberculosis resulting in meningitis, two of whom developed severe brain damage.

Saskatchewan is no longer a leader. On the contrary, in 1987 its largest census area, the northern half of the province, had the highest rate of active new cases of tuberculosis (248.6 per 100,000) of any complete census region in Canada. The situation deteriorated steadily between 1985 and 1987, the number of active cases going up each year from forty-six to fifty-six and then to sixty-three. The Meadow Lake census division has the eighth worst record of the 266 census divisions in Canada and two Indian reserves within it, Buffalo River and Portage la Loche, have rates of 1,000 per 100,000, which is 400 times that of white people in southern Saskatchewan. Although deaths are down since Ferguson's time owing to the availability of effective chemotherapy, and although there are regular outpatient clinics in Fond du Lac, Sandy Bay, Pelican Narrows, Black Lake, Île-à-la-Crosse and La Loche, the present death rate is still unconscionably high. About 20 percent of Métis have tubercle bacilli resistant to antibiotics.

The optimism so evident at the time of Ferguson's retirement has palled. Worldwide, tuberculosis claims three million lives yearly.

George Ferguson! You should be here today.
Saskatchewan needs you: she believes that tuberculosis
Is controlled,
That public health is no longer at risk,
That the province's wealth should be used to acquire luxury.
Wake us up; show us again with your towering wisdom
How to walk the common path of man;
And perform the lowliest task with cheer.

– Vernon Hoeppner, 1989[1]

NOTES

Chapter One

1. Homestead application 7996 for the southeast quarter of section 2 resulted in the issuance of homestead certificate 2786, "established and duly consummated" on 16 November 1891. The same wording was reiterated, using the same application and certificate numbers, in Document 5396, dated 17 December 1897.

2. Only this last mortgage was paid off, on 10 May 1905. On that date, the land titles office listed the value of the 480 acres as $6,350.

3. The northeast quarter of section 16, township 34, range 11, west of the second meridian.

4. The northwest quarter of section 27 was purchased on 30 January 1906 by Hiram McDougall before he married George's sister, Fanny, on 7 August 1907. The southwest quarter of section 27 was purchased by Margaret Jane Ferguson on 6 December 1907, carrying a Canada Permanent mortgage of $1800. In May, 1909, after Hiram sold his quarter to Margaret Jane Ferguson, Mrs. Ferguson negotiated a mortgage on this latter quarter with Imperial Life Assurance for $8,000, though the land was valued at only $2,400. On 16 December 1910, when Vernon was twenty and Frank sixteen, Mrs. Ferguson took another plunge, buying the adjacent farm, the west half of section 23, which carried mortgages totalling $3,950.

Chapter Three

1. England and Wales in 1910, with 1,000 tuberculosis deaths per week, had only 4,000 beds in sixty-one public and twenty-nine private sanatoria.

Chapter Seven

1. Ferguson was also a Fellow of the American College of Chest Physicians,served as president of the Canadian Tuberculosis Association, 1935–36; member of council, American Trudeau Society, 1946–48; member of committee on therapy, American Trudeau Society, 1945–1947; member of Advisory Board, American Trudeau Society, 1948; member of the American Trudeau Society - United States Public Health Service Joint Committee on Immunology, 1948; member of subcommittee on Tuberculin and BCG, World Health Organization, 1948.

2. Christian Smith, in Saskatchewan's "Health Newsletter" *15* (3):2, 15 March 1964.

Chapter Eight

1. Saskatchewan was an exception. "In general the tuberculosis movement neglected rural America." (Teller, 1988).

2. Ferguson had encouraged Dorothy Kline, once her spinal tuberculosis was under control, to attend university. She became a respected professor of biochemistry.

Chapter Nine

1. Hoeppner, V.H., "Invocation to George Ferguson," *Life & Breath* 1 (3):4-5, August 1989 (Saskatchewan Lung Association).

SOURCES

General:

American Review of Tuberculosis, vols. 1–64, 1917–1951.

Bryder, Linda. *Below the Magic Mountain: A Social History of Tuberculosis in Twentieth-Century Britain*. Oxford: Clarendon Press, 1988, 298 pp.

Bulletin of the Canadian Tuberculosis Association, vols. 4–23, 1925–1945.

Larmour, Jean B.D. *A Matter of Life and Breath: The 75 Year History of the Saskatchewan Anti-tuberculosis League and the Saskatchewan Lung Association*. Saskatoon: Saskatchewan Lung Association, 1987.

Proceedings of the Associate Committee on Tuberculosis Research, National Research Council [11 meetings, 1925–1938].

Saskatchewan Anti-tuberculosis League, Minutes, from 1911.

Saskatchewan Anti-tuberculosis League, *The People Versus the White Plague, February 17th, 1911 – February 17th, 1961*.

Smith, E.B. *The Retreat of Tuberculosis, 1850–1950*. London: Croom Helm, 1988.

Teller, M.E. *The Tuberculosis Movement: A Public Health Campaign in the Progressive Era*. New York: Greenwood Press, 1988.

Valley Echo, vols. 1–50, 1918–1969.

Wherrett, G.J. *The Miracle of the Empty Beds*. Toronto: University of Toronto Press.

Chapter 1:

Ferguson family genealogy

Ferguson, R.G. Account book, 1907, 1916, holograph, 10 pp. "George's memories" 9 pp. undated holograph account of boyhood of R.G. Ferguson.

Robert Ferguson (Obituary). *Yorkton Enterprise 10* (10):1, 7, 7 March 1906.

"Ferguson speaks on Father's Life," *Fort Qu'Appelle Times*, December 15, 1981.

Gillan, Welland and Mary, *Followers of the Shield, a Gillan, Geelan Genealogy*, [pp. 145–146 re Frances (Fanny) Hunt who married James F. Ferguson] 1970.
Ferguson, Norma and Robert. "The Ross Family," pp. 502–503 in: Thorlacius, Lillian, *Reflections by the Quills*. Wynyard: Quill Historical Society.
McCullough, A. J. "R.G. Ferguson, '10," *Vox Wesleyana, 14* (6):22–24.
University of Manitoba, Order of Proceedings at the Annual Convocation for Conferring of Degrees, May 12, 1916, and Class and Honor Lists, 1915–1916, p. 75.

Chapter 2:

Seymour, Maurice M. *Valley Echo 10* (2):6, February 1929.
Dr. Maurice Macdonald Seymour (Obituary). *Can. Med. Assoc. J. 20*:212–213, 1929.
"The beginning of anti-tuberculosis work in Saskatchewan." *Valley Echo* 22 (7):17–18, July 1941; 22(8):40–41, 79, Aug. 1941; 22(9):16–18, Sept. 1941; 22(10):16–18, Oct. 1941; 22(11):16–17, Nov. 1941; 22(12):12–15, Dec. 1941.
Saskatchewan Anti-tuberculosis League Minutes (unpublished)
Western Municipal News, vols. *13–25*, 1918–1930.

Chapter 3:

Cowley, Harry R. "I remember." *Valley Echo 37*(1):15, 18, Jan. 1956.
Ferguson, R.G. "The Saskatchewan Sanatorium." *Valley Echo 1*(1):1, Dec. 1919.
Ferguson, R.G. "Something about the *Valley Echo* and its editors." *Valley Echo 21*(12):4–7, 24, Dec. 1940.
Hart, Hazel A. "A patch of the quilt." *Valley Echo 20*(1)12-13, Jan. 1939.
"In Memoriam: Lieut. Col. William Malloch Hart." *Valley Echo 4*(5):7, May 1923.
Johnson, Johanna. "Some of my recollections." *Valley Echo 36*(7):9–14, July 1955.
Mitchell, E.S., "Sanatorium, Fort Qu'Appelle, 1919." *Valley Echo 43*(9):18–19, Sept. 1962.
Mitchell, E.S. "Memories, away back when." *Valley Echo 36*(6):6–8, June 1955.
Walsh, Frank B. "Patients' echoes." *Valley Echo 45*(4):5–6, April 1964.

Chapter 5:

Anonymous. "Tribute to a life's work: Dr. H.C. Boughton." *Valley Echo 40*:2–5, May 1959.
Anonymous. "Amateur hours recreated." *Fort Qu'Appelle Times*, October 1985.
Harvey Crawford Boughton (Obituary). *Can. Med. Assoc. J. 103*:652, 1970.
Cunnings, T.A.J. "Sanatoria in Manitoba." *Valley Echo 26*(1):7–8, Jan. 1945.
Ferguson, Helen. "That a child might live." *Valley Echo 40*(12):4–6, Dec. 1959.

Hart, Hazel A. "How free treatment came to Saskatchewan." *Valley Echo 14*(2):14–15, Feb. 1933.

Hart, Hazel A., "I remember." *Valley Echo 37*(9):2–3, 21–22, Sept. 1956.

Simenson, Vera M. "Tribute to Dr. R.W. Kirkby." *Valley Echo 46*(10):2, 22–23, Oct. 1965.

Stubbings, W.J. *A History of the Associated Canadian Travellers, Yorkton Club, 1933–1983*, pp. 1–8, 29–34.

Zdunich, Darlene J. "Tuberculosis and World War One Veterans," M.A. thesis, Department of History, University of Calgary, 1984, 182 pp.

Chapter 6:

Andrews, C.H. "League services take wings." *Valley Echo 16*(5):10–11, May 1935.

Anonymous. "First inhabitants of Qu'Appelle Valley honour Dr. R.G. Ferguson. *Valley Echo 16*(6):10–11, June 1935.

Anonymous. "Indian baby clinic." *Valley Echo 7*(7):15, July 1926 and7(8):14, Aug. 1926.

Anonymous. "Associate Committee on Tuberculosis." 3-page typescript, History Collection, CISTI Library, Ottawa.

Associate Committee on Medical Research. "Assisted research grants." Ottawa, February 1940.

Associate Committee on Medical Research. Proceedings of the second through sixteenth meetings, 1938–1945.

Ettinger, G.H. "History of the Associate Committee on Medical Research, Ottawa, 1938–1946," 5 pp.

Ferguson, R.G. "Journal on a trip to Portage La Loche," typescript, 13 pp.

Frappier, Armand. Letter to R.G. Ferguson, 13 October 1933.

"Grants authorized by the Associate Committee on Medical Research in 1939–40 and Applications for 1940–41." 1-page typescript, Banting Collection, Vol. *5*, CISTI Library, Ottawa.

"Grants in aid of Research awarded by the National Research Council, 1947–1948," pp. 1, 12.

Maher, S.J. "Tuberculosis among the American Indians." *Am. Rev. Tuberculosis 19*:407–411, 1929.

Marshall, I.B. "The evolution of the National Research Council of Canada's policy on support of postgraduate science training and research in Canadian Universities," term paper for Professor R. Murray, School of Public Administration, Queen's University. [Contains summary of annual research grants]

McGibony, J.R., and Dahlstrom, A.W. "Tuberculosis among Montana Indians." *Am. Review Tuberculosis 52*:104–121, 1945.

Motherwell, Patricia. "Under the T.B. Cross," pp. 303–305 in *Dance on the Bridge, a History of the Abernethy Area*, Abernethy Historical Association, 1983.

National Research Council. Report of the President. [Yearly from 1924–25 through 1950].

Panel on Tuberculosis of the Associate Committee on Medical Research, National Research Council, thirteenth meeting, 14 January 1946, pp. 1–2.

Phillipson, D.J.C. "Associate Committees of the National Research Council of Canada, 1917–1975," pp. 26, 78–79. Ottawa: National Research Council, 1983.

"Research Grants, 1946–1951". Awards Office, Administration and Personnel, National Research Council, 20 September 1951, p. 77.

Thistle, Mel. *The Inner Ring: The Early History of the National Research Council of Canada*, pp. 166–167, 216, 285–288. Toronto: University of Toronto Press, 1966.

Walker, J.R. "Tuberculosis among the Oglala Sioux Indians." *Am. J. Med. Sci. 132*:600–605, 1906.

"War History of the Associate Committees of the National Research Council." Q. Panel on Tuberculosis, pp. 118–119.

Chapter 7

Anonymous. "Towards better health for all." *Valley Echo 36*(5):6, May 1955.

Anonymous. "Bovine Tuberculosis." *Valley Echo 34*(6):1–2, June 1953.

Anonymous. "New fluorographic unit purchased." *Valley Echo 26*(8):33, Aug. 1945.

Anonymous. "Too much chest x-ray?" *Valley Echo 38*(11):3, Nov. 1957.

Anonymous. "The League's first mass survey." *Valley Echo 48*(1&2):14, Jan–Feb. 1967.

Callin, Gertrude. "Nursing students at Saskasan." *Valley Echo* 43(12):11, 23, 1962.

Callin, Gertrude. "A plea for nursing education in tuberculosis." *Valley Echo 45*(9), Sept. 1964.

Connell, R.S. "The story of x-rays." *Valley Echo 23*(1):6–8, Jan. 1942.

Connell, R.S. "Fluorography." *Valley Echo 23*(6):6–7, June 1942.

de Abreu, Manoel. "The bearers of shadows." *Diseases of the Chest 11*:639–647, 1945.

Lee, Edith. "Nurses' Aides in Saskatchewan." *Valley Echo 30*(6):4, 1949.

Van Allen, Willard W. "Protecting photofluorographic personnel from excessive radiation." *Public Health Reports 65*:865–868, 7 July 1950.

Chapter 8

Anonymous. "Sorrowing thousands mourn loved doctor." *Yorkton Enterprise 69*(9):4 March 1964, pp. 1, 7, 8.

Brock, Veronica Eddy. *The Valley of Flowers: A Story of a TB Sanatorium*. Moose Jaw: Coteau Books, 1988.

Boughton, H.C. "Doctor Robert George Ferguson, an appreciation." *Valley Echo* 45(6):2–3, 23, June 1964.

Dempsey, H.A. *History in Their Blood: The Indian Portraits of Nicholas de Grandmaison*. Vancouver: Douglas & McIntyre, 1982. 124 pp.

Ferguson, Norma. "Helen Josephine (Ross) Ferguson." Typescript.

Ferguson, R.G. "My God." Typescript, April 1948.

"Mrs. Margaret J. Ferguson entered into rest." *Yorkton Enterprise*, Jan. 22, 1949.

Fallis, Margaret Ferguson, and Motherwell, Patricia Ferguson. Audio tape of reminiscences, 4 August 1984 (transcribed by CSH).

Froh, Frank [Tribute]. *Valley Echo* 45(3):6–7, March 1964.

Kirkby, R.W. "Dr. George Ferguson, our Operational Founder." *Valley Echo* 45(3):7–8, 23, March 1964.

Roberts, R.D. "An Employee's Tribute." *Valley Echo* 45(3):17–18, March 1964.

Seymour, Margaret R. "Fort San's 'Unforgettable Character': Alf Johnson." *Valley Echo* 45(4):10–11, 20, April 1964.

Smith-Windsor, T. "Links with our past." *Medscan 1*:4–6, 1986 (University of Saskatchewan College of Medicine).

Stewart, D.A. "Tuberculosis problems of Today." *Am. Rev. Tuberculosis* 4: 1-11, 1920.

Wherrett, G.J. "R.G. Ferguson, O.B.E., B.A., M.D., LL.D., an appreciation." *Canadian Medical Association Journal 90*:995–996, 1964.

———. "Tribute." *Valley Echo* 45(3):4–5, March 1964.

Chapter 9

Grzybowski, Stefan. "Tuberculosis, a look at the world situation." *Chest 84*:756–761, 1983.

Styblo, Karei. "Overview and epidemiologic assessment of the current global tuberculosis situation with an emphasis on control in developing countries." *Reviews of Infectious Diseases 11*, Suppl. 2, S339–S346, 1989.

APPENDICES

Appendix I

A. Publications by Robert George Ferguson

Cook, A.B., Ferguson, R.G., Cairns, J.F., and R.H. Brighton. *Report of the Saskatchewan Anti-tuberculosis Commission.* Regina: JW Reid, King's Printer, 1922.

Ferguson, R.G. A tuberculosis survey of 1,346 school children in Saskatchewan. *Can. Med. Assoc. J. 12*:381–383, 1922.

———. The differentiation and treatment of lung abscess by exploratory pulmonary puncture and bismuth injection. *Can. Med Assoc. J. 14*:597–603, 1924.

———. Medical examination of school children. *Can. Med. Assoc. J. 15*:397–399, 1925.

———. The most important agencies in a provincial campaign against tuberculosis. *Can. Med. Assoc. J. 15*:799–803, 1925.

———. Follow-up information on 1,747 tuberculosis patients one to seven years after discharge from a sanatorium. *Am. Rev. Tuberculosis 14*:625-645, 1926.

———. A pure milk supply for the farm home. *[Can.] Publ. Health J. 18*:151–155, 1927.

———. Tuberculosis among the Indians of the great Canadian plains. *Trans. Nat. Assoc. Prev. Tuberculosis*, London, *14*:5–56, 1928. Reprinted London: Adlard & Son.

———. Study of epidemiology of tuberculosis in primitive people. *Edinburgh Med. J. 36*:199–206, 1929.

———. The Indian tuberculosis problem and some preventive measures. *Trans. Nat. Tuberculosis Assoc.*, Toronto, 93–106, 1933. *Can. Med. Assoc. J. 30*:544–547, 1934.

———. Some light thrown on infection, resistance and segregation by a study of tuberculosis among Indians. *Trans. Am. Clin. Climatolog. Assoc. 50*:18–26, 1934.

———. Activities in a province-wide programme for the control of tuberculosis. *Can. Public Health J. 26*:130–137, 1935.

McNeill, J.W., and R.G. Ferguson. *Survey of Tuberculosis in Mental Institutions in*

Saskatchewan, 1929–1935. Regina: Department of Public Health, 1936.

Ferguson, R.G. Some simple observations and procedures of assistance to the practitioner in the diagnosis and eradication of tuberculosis. *Can. Med. Assoc. J. 32*:524–528, 1935.

———. Tuberculosis among nurses. *Can. Nurse 32*:545–548, 1936.

———. Address by the president. *Bull. Can. Tuberculosis Assn. 15*:15–17, 1936.

———. President's address. *Bull. Can. Tuberculosis Assn. 16*:1–3,8–9, 1937.

———. In memoriam: David Alexander Stewart. *J. Thorac. Surg. 7*:458, 1938.

———. Some fundamentals in tuberculosis prevention. *Can. Publ. Health J. 29*:203–212, 1938.

Dobbie, W.J., Hatfield, W.H., Baker, A.H., Ferguson, R.G., Ross, E.L., Brink, G.C., Gregoire, G., Collins, R.J., Campbell, P.S., Creelman, P.A., and G.J. Wherrett. *Programme for an Intensive Community Campaign against Tuberculosis.* Ottawa: Canadian Tuberculosis Association.

Ferguson, R.G. Protection of unavoidably exposed persons against tuberculosis. *Journal-Lancet 60*:170–173, 1940.

———. David A. Stewart memorial lecture: changes in the epidemiological conception of tuberculosis. *University of Manitoba Medical Journal 13*:62–68, February 1942.

———. Recent advances in tuberculosis control. *Can. J. Publ. Health 35*:109–112, 1944.

———. Recent advances in the campaign against tuberculosis. *Am. Rev. Tuberculosis 50*:131–135, 1944.

———. BCG vaccination in hospitals and sanatoria of Saskatchewan. *Am. Rev. Tuberculosis 54*:325–339, 1946. *Can. J. Publ. Health 37*:435–451,1946. *Boll. Med. Social Santiago 14*:238–250, 1947.

———. and A.B. Simes. BCG vaccination of Indian infants in Saskatchewan. *Tubercle 30*:5–11, 1949.

———. Provisions for the prevention and care of tuberculosis in Canada. *Med. J. Australia 2*:768–771, 1949. *Can. Med. Assoc. J. 62*:131–135, 1950.

———. *Studies in Tuberculosis.* Toronto: University of Toronto Press. 1955.

B. Papers by Other Members of Staff

Anderson, H.J. A study of 345 family contacts with tuberculous lesions. *Can. Publ. Health J.* 32:594–600, 1941.

Andrews, C.H. Cerebral air embolism complicating articial pneumothorax. Report of a case. *Am. Rev. Tuberculosis* 23:435–439, 1931.

———. Bronchial stenosis in pulmonary tuberculosis. *Can.Med.Assoc. J.* 33:36–41, 1935.

———. First steps in pneumolysis. *Am. Rev. Tuberculosis* 33:36–43, 1936.

———. Thorascopic removal of broken aspirating needle: case report. *J. Thorac. Surg.* 6:456–457, 1937.

———. Closed intrapleural pneumonolysis. Report of 124 cases. *Can Med. Assoc J.* 40:548-553, 1941.

Barclay, W.S. A study of tuberculosis contacts in families. *Am. Rev. Tuberculosis* 26:192–208, 1932.

———. A review of Thoracoplasties in Saskatchewan. *Can. Med. Assoc. J.* 45:525-529, 1941.

Barnett, G.D. Results of mass surveys in the province of Saskatchewan, 1942-1947. *Can. Tuberculosis Assoc. Med Papers*, fiftieth annual meeting, 33–36,1950.

Bennett, C.F. Tuberculosis in recent immigrants. *Can. Publ. Health J.* 31:515–530, 1940.

Boughton, H.C. New case finding in tuberculosis: methods used in the rural province of Saskatchewan. *Can. Publ. Health J.* 28:259–264, 1937.

Kirkby, R.W. Unusual termination in a case of tuberculous spine. *Can. Med. Assoc. J.* 31:64, 1934.

———. An early sign in tuberculous meningitis. *Can. Med. Assoc. J.* 31:415, 1934.

———. Discovery of cases of active tuberculosis amongst ex-patients in rural province. *Can. Publ. Health J.* 28:10–12, 1937.

Molony, I.C. A study of 1,000 cases of adult tuberculosis and its bearing on diagnosis. *Am. Rev. Tuberculosis* 19:99–118, 1929.

Simes, A.B., and L.E. Paynter. A study of the occurrence of virulent tubercle bacilli in excreta of tuberculous Indian children. *Tubercle* 15:498–503, 1934.

Wherrett, G.J. Follow-up information on 2,031 tuberculosis patients one to thirteen years after discharge from Sanatoria. *Am. Rev. Tuberculosis* 31:62–73, 1935.

Appendix II

Family Lists

CHILDREN OF ROBERT AND AND MARGARET JANE (FISHER) FERGUSON
(R.G. FERGUSON AND HIS SIBLINGS)

The oldest son of James Ferguson's second family, Robert Ferguson, married Margaret Jane Fisher (7 June 1855 – 21 January 1948) in Bervie, Ontario on 15 July 1874. There were 16 children:

1. Thomas Francis. Born 22 August 1875 at Ripley, Ont.
   Died accidentally in April 1887 at Joliette, N.D.
2. Emma Eliza [Eliza]. Born 8 July 1877 at Ripley, Ont.
   Married George Muir at Joliette, N.D. on 4 November 1896.
   Died 1960.
3. William James [Jim]. Born 7 October 1879 at Ripley, Ont.
   Married Elspeth Agnes Emerson at Pembina, N.D. on 3 August 1904.
   Died 23 August 1955 at Seattle, Wash. Four children.
4. Ida May. Born 15 November 1881 at Joliette, N.D.
   Died 1902, of tuberculosis, at Joliette, N.D.
5. Ida May's twin, stillborn.
6. **Robert George**. Born 12 September 1883 at Joliette, N.D.
   Married Helen F.J. Ross on 5 July 1916 at Wynyard, Sask.
   Died 1 March 1964 at Regina, Sask.
   [Seven children and their progeny will be listed separately]
7. Fanny Amelia. Born 23 May 1885 at Joliette, N.D.
   Married 7 August 1907 at Yorkton to Hiram Marcus McDougall.
   Three children. Died 3 March 1986 at Saskatoon, Sask.
8. Thomas Fisher. Born 2 May 1887 at Joliette, N.D.
   Married 18 September 1912 at Yorkton to Susan Alice Christie.
   Died 25 November 1964 at North Battleford, Sask. Five children.
9. Laura Mabelle. Born 27 October 1888 at Joliette, N.D.
   Married Melzar Ross Ruttle on 1 January 1929.
   Died 14 November 1973 at Yorkton, Sask. One adopted child.
10. Vernon Stewart. Born 14 February 1890 at Joliette, N.D.
    Married 17 December 1917 at Toronto to Norma Fern Rogers.
    Died 13 July 1930 at Yorkton, Sask. Two sons.
11. Herby Wesley. Born 9 February 1891 at Joliette, N.D. Died of diphtheria at Joliette, N.D. in 1901.

12. Clara Myrtle. Born 9 May 1892 at Joliette, N.D.
    Married 5 December 1918 at Yorkton, Sask. to William Henry Richardson. Three children. Died 18 March 1980.
13. Frank William. Born 9 February 1894 at Joliette, N.D. Died 1916 in wartime service in Belgium. Unmarried. No children.
14. Etta Pearl. Born 9 December 1895 at Joliette, N.D.
    Married 8 February 1916 at Yorkton to William Ewart Greenfield. Three children. Died 26 February 1978 at Vancouver, B.C.
15. Helen Evangeline. Born 18 September 1900 at Joliette, N.D.
    Married Arthur Percy Swallow on 20 May 1922 at Yorkton, Sask. Two children. Died 10 December 1974 at Weyburn, Sask.
16. Margaret Victoria. Born 30 April 1902 at Joliette, N.D.
    Married William Selkirk Clegg at Winnipeg on 31 May 1923. Four children. Died 1 September 1965 at Edmonton.

The Children and Grandchildren of Helen and Robert George Ferguson

Robert George Ferguson was married 5 July 1916 at Wynyard, Sask. to Helen Florence Josephine Ross, born 3 February 1892 at Burford, Ontario to Mr. and Mrs. Thomas Hervey Ross. [Helen died 8 February 1983 at Fort Qu'Appelle, Saskatchewan].

1. Robert Ross Ferguson, born 13 May 1917 at Winnipeg, Man.
   Married 7 June 1946 to Norma Cecelia Johnson of Battrum,Sask.
   Four children:
   - Robert Martin, born 13 April 1948 at Saskatoon.
   - Norma Laurell [Laura], born 18 January 1950 at Qu'Appelle.
   - George Mitchell, born 19 May 1952 at Qu'Appelle.
   - Colleen Helen, born 14 October 1958 at Qu'Appelle.
2. Helen Elliott Ferguson [Honey], born 4 October 1918 at Fort Qu'Appelle. Died at Yorkton, 4 August 1964.
   Married 8 September 1941 to Robert Bedford Hart.
   Three children:
   - David Bedford, born 29 June 1944.
   - Helen Candis [Candy], born 27 February 1949.
   - Royland George [George], born 29 September 1951.
3. Margaret Fisher Ferguson, Born 10 March 1920.
   Married Major John Love [who was killed on "D" Day, 6 June 1944].
   No children.

Married Wing/Commander Keith Fallis [who drowned in New Zealand, 8 March 1980].
Four children:
   Penelopy Helen, born 21 June 1947.
   David George, born 7 May 1949.
   Cynthia Margaret, born 7 April 1951.
   Robert Millard, born 11 August 1952.

4. Mary Patricia [Pat], born 15 December 1921 at Fort Qu'Appelle.
Married Richard Motherwell 10 July 1943 [he died 9 September 1953]. Three children:
   Roberta Flynne [Shera], born 9 July 1944.
   Shannon Laura, born 18 August 1949.
   Richard Stephney [Dickie], born 21 February 1953.
Second marriage to George Dyck, June 1991.

5. Sheelagh Josephine, born 24 March 1924.
Married Gordon Henry Barrable on 7 May 1948.
Four children:
   Sheelagh Ann [Shee-Ann], born 23 October 1949.
   Sterling Ross [Ross], born 12 August 1951.
   Robert Gordon, born 2 July 1953.
   William McLean, born 12 January 1961.

6. John Vincent, born 24 March 1924 (twin of Sheelagh).
Died 9 December 1925.

7. David George Ferguson, born 23 December 1925.
Married June Lyn Evelyn on 12 May 1950.
Four children:
   Leah-Anne, born 15 March 1951.
   David Lloyd [Lloyd], born 17 September 1954.
   Jill Lynda, born 16 September 1956.
   Michael Patrick, born 16 November 1964.
Second marriage to Dora Fryer.

Appendix III

R.G. Ferguson's Accomplishments

R.G. Ferguson's extraordinary efforts contributed to a number of breakthroughs in the early detection and treatment of tuberculosis in North America:

- First school survey for tuberculosis
- First universally free tuberculosis treatment
- First statistically controlled BCG prophylaxis in Indian infants
- First BCG prophylaxis in student nurses
- First community-wide photofluorographic lung survey
- First jurisdiction with sufficent beds for TB patients

INDEX

ENVIRONMENTAL CHOICE · CHOIX ENVIRONNEMENTAL ·

Printed on paper
containing over 50%
recycled paper including
10% post-consumer fibre.

Printed in Canada